Reframing Mental Health
in Schools

Reframing Mental Health in Schools

Using Case Stories to Promote Global Dialogue

Erin Keith and Kimberly Maich

ROWMAN & LITTLEFIELD
Lanham • Boulder • New York • London

Published by Rowman & Littlefield
An imprint of The Rowman & Littlefield Publishing Group, Inc.
4501 Forbes Boulevard, Suite 200, Lanham, Maryland 20706
www.rowman.com

86-90 Paul Street, London EC2A 4NE, United Kingdom

British Library Cataloguing in Publication Information Available

Library of Congress Cataloging-in-Publication Data

Names: Keith, Erin, 1971- author. | Maich, Kimberly, 1969- author.
Title: Reframing mental health in schools : using case stories to promote global dialogue / Erin Keith, Kimberly Maich.
Description: Lanham : Rowman & Littlefield, [2022] | Includes bibliographical references. | Summary: "The book includes first-hand stories and experiences collaborating with school teams as they work with, support and program for students from around the globe displaying a wide variety of mental health concerns"— Provided by publisher.
Identifiers: LCCN 2022011977 (print) | LCCN 2022011978 (ebook) | ISBN 9781475852875 (cloth) | ISBN 9781475852882 (paperback) | ISBN 9781475852899 (epub)
Subjects: LCSH: Students—Mental health—Case studies. | School environment— Psychological aspects—Case studies. | School improvement programs—Case studies. | Students with social disabilities—Education—Case studies.
Classification: LCC LB3430 .K45 2022 (print) | LCC LB3430 (ebook) | DDC 371.7/13—dc23/eng/20220511
LC record available at https://lccn.loc.gov/2022011977
LC ebook record available at https://lccn.loc.gov/2022011978

Contents

Preface

Reframing Mental Health in Schools: Using Case Stories to Promote Global Dialogue is about "lifting up" the voices of students in kindergarten to Grade 12 who have experienced mental health distress from various countries around the globe.

According to the OECD (2021), children's mental well-being has been significantly impacted by the current COVID-19 pandemic, due to prolonged at-home learning mandates, a disruption in mental health support services, and a weakening of the protective factors such as daily routine and connection with invested partners including teachers, educational assistants, family members, and community agencies. Even prior to the pandemic, children's well-being was worsening due to students' uptake of digital technologies and access to social media (OECD, 2021). Mental health literacy was being prioritized in education in some countries with a wraparound model of school-based supports offered to some degree. However, many countries around the globe still face barriers and stigma related to understanding and supporting students' mental health.

This book serves to offer global stories of students' well-being experiences and invites readers to engage in rich dialogue that intersects culture, race, access, and even barriers to supports. These student stories espouse mental health-related concerns such as anxiety, depression, eating disorders, and suicidal ideations and outline inclusive strategies school staff can facilitate and scaffold with students that build their resiliency, social-emotional/healthy relationship skills, and support their healthy healing and a path toward recovery.

REFERENCES

OECD. (2021). Supporting young people's mental health through the COVID-19 crisis. OECD Policy Brief. https://www.oecd.org/coronavirus/policy-responses/supporting-young-people-s-mental-health-through-the-covid-19-crisis-84e143e5/.

Acknowledgments

Erin: What a transformative journey this book partnership has been for me! Thank you to my wildly supportive coauthor, Dr. Kimberly Maich, for bringing our vision to life in innumerable ways, including your incredible academic contacts, and to our gifted book contributors for sharing stories about your students while weaving in your own lived experiences. I express my sincere gratitude. My work in K–12 education as a teacher has propelled my motivation to "lift up" the voices of my students who are brave, sincere, and courageous and who are woven into heart. Lastly, to my biggest fans, my loving family, Stephen, Avery, Megan, Cassie, Ginger, and our band of furry pets: thank you for filling me with joy and fire.

Kimberly: I would like to thank my coauthor Dr. Erin Keith for leading this project, our research assistants funded through Memorial University, and our wonderfully passionate and dedicated case story contributors from around the globe. My family is foundational to any work that I do; thank you to John, Robert, Grace, Hannah, and Quincey for being that foundation and for teaching me about mental health along the way.

Introduction: Overview and Significance

Current statistics in Canada show that one in five students experience mental health issues (Canada, 2012; CAMH, 2021). Mental health disorders cause significant distress, impairing students' wholistic functioning at school, at home, and in the community (Children's Mental Health Ontario, 2014). Research has shown that prevention and early intervention strategies targeting students at risk for mental health stressors are beneficial, cost effective, and reduce the need for costlier, intensive interventions (Ontario Ministry of Education, 2013; CAMH, 2021). Since students spend most of their day at school, schools are obliged to play an important role in the prevention and early intervention of students' mental health needs (Durlak & Wells, 2011).

From an international perspective, mental health-related issues cannot be ignored. Children's mental health is an issue without borders, and it is increasingly becoming an epidemic, especially since the onset of the COVID-19 pandemic. According to United Nations Foundation (UNF, 2021), the prevalence of mental health diagnoses has peaked in the Middle East, North Africa, North America, and Western Europe (para. 8). In addition, the global statistics are bleak with "89 million adolescent boys aged 10-19 and 77 million adolescent girls aged 10-19 live with a mental disorder—40% of them anxiety and/or depression" (UNF, 2021, para. 8). Unfortunately, these statistics are only for those children who are fortunate to receive medical supports and a diagnosis. What about those children who do *not* have access to medical supports or who are ignored due to the persistent stigma associated with mental health? As alarming as the diagnostic statistics are, they represent only a small fraction of the real data. Mental health *IS* health, and global societies can no longer shame nor stigmatize children for voicing their needs and calls for help (UNF, 2021).

The purpose of this case stories book is to present unique narratives of international students from K–Grade 12 who are experiencing various types of mental health stressors, some of which are diagnosed and others that are not. Our respected and esteemed case study contributors bring their lived experiences supporting, caring, and advocating for students in a wellness capacity from countries including Canada, France, Iran, Argentina, West Africa, New Zealand, Croatia, and more. We also have included a story of an Indigenous student, PHOENIX, who experiences mental health trauma due to exposure to long-standing intergenerational and historical traumas experienced by PHOENIX's Peoples.

The significance of this case stories book is to permit more courageous conversations between preservice teachers, educators, support staff, and administration alongside parents and community members. The authentic, lived experiences of children and youth "must be acknowledged, listened to, and taken seriously by the adults in their lives" (UNF, 2021, para. 12). As a nurturing and caring society, the mental health of youth must be protected both at home and at school, regardless of where they live in the world. We hope these case studies can (re)frame the stigma that still exists in many cultures and prioritize that mental health is indeed health.

Yours in Action, Care, and Advocacy,
Erin Keith, EdD, OCT and Kimberly Maich,
PhD, OCT, BCBA-D, R Psych, C Psych

Section 1

ELEMENTARY (K–6)
SECTION OVERVIEW

In elementary schools, mental health stressors in children under age twelve are underdiagnosed and are often masked by internalized behaviors such as worry, fear, social withdrawal, somatic complaints, or by externalized behaviors such as aggression, rule breaking, vandalism, and poor impulse control (Harvard University, 2021). From a school-based perspective, it is never too late to support young children with mental health coping strategies and early interventions. Although prevention is key, with the nurturing support of stable and responsive caregivers, teachers, family members, and school-based, trauma-informed interventions, young children can be protected from further harm and aided in developing lasting coping skills to overcome their psychological adversity and possibly restore their wellness (Harvard University, 2021).

In this Elementary K–Grade 6 section, we learn about a six-year-old Black student (Keshawn) whose mother is experiencing depression herself and the impact it is having on Keshawn's school experiences (Case Story #1: Navigating Early Years Wellness as a Young Black Male Student; contributor Erin Keith). In this case, a socio-ecological lens centered on building relational connections between family and school partners is used to support both mother and her son while honoring their Jamaican culture and heritage. Case Story #2 is entitled "Embracing Body Diversity to Prevent Eating Disorders in a Classroom Setting in Canada" (contributor Margaret Janse van Rensburg). This case discusses the authentic conversations needed in school by teachers related to body diversity and healthy eating. Morgan, age eleven, is a female student who has recently begun to take diet pills due to pressures from social media and peers. We are introduced to the Health At Every Size® (HAES®) model, a whole class approach to discuss weight bias and stigma related to body size while ensuring Morgan's privacy.

In Case Story #3 (Autism and Anxiety in a Primary School-Aged Child in France), contributors Mélissa Villella and Hélène Abdelnour introduce us to Zoe, a five-year-old from France who has both autism and anxiety. Here we learn the value of family-school relationships and centering Zoe's voice and mother's knowledge about her daughter. This powerful triad of parent–child–school ensures that Zoe is supported to better manage her anxiety and succeed in primary school both academically and socially/emotionally. For the next two cases, we travel to West Africa to learn about the stigma related to mental health and the measures these societies are prioritizing for young students and the role families play. Although much more is needed from a destigmatization and funding perspective, strong teacher advocates and school personnel such as social workers, are leading the way for change (Case Story #4: Assisting a Student with Bipolar Disorder in West Africa; contributors Margaret Janse van Rensburg and Olivia Atsin; and Case Story #5: "Being My Neighbor's Keeper": Mental Health Challenges in Ghana; contributors Magnus Mfoafo-M'Carthy and Jennie Beck). In Case Story #6 entitled "How Reading Gaps Impact a Young Child's Wellness in Canada" (contributor Jeffrey MacCormack), we learn about Sophia's self-perceptions that she is "not a reader" and the impact it has on her well-being. With specific reading interventions in place and open communication with family, Sophia's view of herself as a reader is strengthened. Lastly, we end this section with PHOENIX, an Indigenous grade 5 learner who is forced to attend the local colonial public school (Case Story #7—PHOENIX: An Indigenous Learner; contributor Gus Hill). In this case, Dr. Hill shares both the history and present experiences of Aboriginal Peoples in Canada who have endured innumerable years of intergenerational trauma, racism, and erasure of language, culture, land, resources, and children. Through PHOENIX's story, we learn the importance of relational engagement, promoting diversity, and being cognizant of white privilege within colonial structures such as elementary schools. We are urged to dismantle these prevalent notions and examine our own worldviews so that children like PHOENIX can begin to trust, heal, learn, and thrive as their authentic, wholistic selves.

We encourage you to "sit in a space" that is both reflective (e.g., in dialogue with others) and reflexive (e.g., in dialogue with self). These case studies are crafted to evoke a wide range of emotions, and sometimes discomfort, in an effort to promote courageous conversations, action, and reconciliation. Children's mental health can be more positively shaped by how responsive, caring, and relational our actions are toward them. Sometimes we are their sole "advocate" and "trusted person." It is a role that carries immense weight. We are not intended to be their "heroes," but we can certainly offer supportive, nurturing conditions within schools for them to restore, heal, and eventually soar on their own.

REFERENCES

Canada Newswire. (2012, June 1). The Council of Ontario Directors of Education releases paper on Children's Mental Health. *Canada Newswire.* http://www.newswire.ca/en/story/985211/the-public-council-of-ontario-directors-of-education-releases-paper-on-children-s-mental-health.

Children's Mental Health Ontario (CAMH). (2014). *Just the facts.* http://www.kidsmentalhealth.ca/join_the_cause/just_the_facts.php.

Children's Mental Health Ontario (CAMH). (2021). *Teacher resources.* https://cmho.org/teacher-resources/.

Durlak, J. A., & Wells, A. M. (2011). Evaluation of indicated preventative intervention (secondary-prevention) mental health programs for children and adolescents. *School Mental Health, 3*(4), 191–208. https://doi.org/10.1023/A:1022162015815.

Harvard University. (2021). *Early childhood mental health.* Center on the Developing Child. https://developingchild.harvard.edu/science/deep-dives/mental-health/.

Ontario Ministry of Education. (2013). *Supporting minds: An educator's guide to promoting students' mental health and well-being.* http://www.edu.gov.on.ca/eng/document/reports/SupportingMinds.pdf.

United Nations Foundation (UNF). (2021). *We can't fail another generation: 5 Things to know about child and adolescent mental health.* Global Health. https://unfoundation.org/blog/post/we-cant-fail-another-generation-5-things-to-know-about-child-and-adolescent-mental-health/.

Chapter 1

Case Story #1—Navigating Early Years Wellness as a Young Black Male Student

Erin Keith

THEORETICAL MODEL AND BACKGROUND

For the following case study of Keshawn, age six, Black male in a Grade 1 mainstream classroom, a socio-ecological model of mental health understanding situates the dialogue of this case study. A socio-ecological model recognizes the dynamic interrelatedness among social and environmental factors, including the family, school, community, and mental health supports as developed by Bronfenbrenner (1977). This integrative model is based on a collectivist orientation of supports (i.e., family, extended caregivers, community, school) that centers the child and family through a metaphoric lens of "it takes a village." The model also acknowledges the rich cultural traditions of the family and although the family would be considered at-risk in terms of socioeconomic status, the relational nature of the model reorientates the family's social ecology from "at-risk" to "at-hope" (Henderson et al., 2016).

FAMILY BACKGROUND OF KESHAWN

Keshawn is a racialized student with a Jamaican cultural heritage. His mother is the primary parent and caregiver, and he has no siblings. Keshawn was born in Ontario in a large, suburban city. His mother, born in Jamaica, works part time at the local grocery store while Keshawn is at school. They live in subsidized housing, walking some distance to Keshawn's school. Keshawn's mother does not have access to a car and relies on extended family and friends for transportation needs or on public transit. Keshawn is quite young and is one of the youngest children in his Grade 1 class. He has had a history of well-being concerns since kindergarten, as voiced by his mom and school team. He rarely shows positive emotions, has difficulty connecting with his peers, and is often a distant observer in the classroom. Sometimes this lack of connection is externalized with more aggressive behaviors (e.g., hitting, biting, and pulling hair) of peers and some children in his class have voiced they are "afraid" of Keshawn. Although Keshawn has been seen by a family doctor, no formal diagnosis has been made. Keshawn is awaiting an appointment with a child psychiatrist and presently is not taking any medications. His mother has shared with the school administrators that she has mental health issues herself, including depression which she feels impacts her parenting abilities. Community support agencies such as Children's Aid Society have serviced the family on and off for several years, and Keshawn's family is on the wait-list for in-home parenting support. Keshawn does not see his biological father and does not have a caring male figure in his life, presently. Due to his mother's ongoing mental health issues, Keshawn's attendance at school is not consistent. If Keshawn is aggressive toward peers or adults at school and she is called to pick him up, his mother will often keep Keshawn home the next day or two.

KESHAWN'S STORY

The bell rings, and I take a deep breath as I walk down the hall to meet my students. Keshawn had a difficult day on Friday. Keshawn's mother was called to pick him up early because he shoved the special education teacher in the stomach. Keshawn did not want to put his food away when he was asked to do. Keshawn then did not attend school yesterday. His mother said she was keeping him home when the school secretary called to check in but said he would be back on Tuesday. I hope we have a positive entry to the day because Keshawn's entry into school often sets the tone for the rest of the day. As I round the corner of the hallway, I can see the school behavior teaching assistant (BTA) walking swiftly after a student with her walkie-talkie in hand. I did not get a good glimpse of the student, but it seems he had come inside before the rest of the class was ready to be picked up and was now running through the school. As I open the door to go outside and greet my Grade 1 students, I am told by three colleagues that Keshawn is in the school running around. My heart sinks. I really wanted to connect with Keshawn this morning and let him know that today is a fresh, new day.

As I walk my students to our classroom, I see Keshawn. He takes one step toward me and then turns around and runs upstairs. The school's BTA and the vice-principal are following him from a safe distance. I can hear the VP on the walkie-talkie updating our school's principal and special education teacher about Keshawn's situation. We have a safety plan for Keshawn that outlines staff response should Keshawn demonstrate specific behaviors, such as running out of class, throwing objects or furniture and not complying with staff requests after repeated requests. I know my role in this situation is to stay with my students and carry on with the day. Hopefully, Keshawn will calm and be able to come to class.

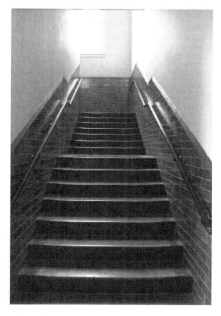

Figure 1.1 Beginning the day. Case Story #1. *iStock—Standard License.* https://stock.adobe.com/ca/images/light-hits-dark-stairwell-of-old-nineteenth-century-school-house-in-england-with-hanging-light-burgundy-red-tiles-and-shiny-black-painted-stairs/144989259?prev_url=detail.

We have worked hard as a school team to recognize Keshawn's triggers and put into place some coping strategies such as a calming space in the classroom to help him self-regulate, a home-school communication booklet for the mother to ask how his night/morning was before school, some hands-on discovery activities using Kinetic sand, Play-Doh, 2D tile blocks, and other building manipulatives. I have noticed Keshawn enjoys going to his calming space even when he is not escalated, and he likes the independent learning activities. I have added materials to the calming space that are culturally diverse (e.g., picture books, skin color crayons, etc.)

BRIEF CRITICAL RESPONSE QUESTIONS

1. Browse through online examples of calming spaces. What other names can you find for this type of environmental strategy for self-regulation (e.g., cozy corner)?
2. How might you change Keshawn's entry to avoid him running through the school and make it a more successful experience?
3. Find and describe an example of a culturally responsive picture book related to self-regulation or another social-emotional-behavioral topic that you might include in the calming space.

REFLECTIVE RESPONSE QUESTIONS

1. Keshawn arrives at your door fifteen minutes after you last saw him running in the hallway. The school BTA lets you know he is "ready" to come into the classroom. You look at Keshawn and he appears calm. What do you do next that supports a socio-ecological model? Support your reasoning.
2. Name, describe, and explain two other culturally responsive elements you would add to Keshawn's support program. Rationalize your choices with support from peer-reviewed literature.
3. Name, describe, and explain one or two elements you would remove from Keshawn's support program. Support your choices.
4. How do you foster and repair relationships in the classroom between Keshawn and his peers, some who are quite fearful of him?
5. As Keshawn's teacher, how do you (re)frame colleagues' and other community members' (lunchroom supervisors, parent volunteers, etc.) view of Keshawn as "at-risk" to "at-hope" in an authentic, equitable, anti-racist, and relational manner?

Strategies of support to consider:

- Visuals of the calming space and discovery activities
- Connect with colleagues to consult on the co-development of a safety plan
- Home-school communication book
- Data-tracking sheets (ABC chart, frequency chart, etc.)
- Picture books on the topic of student "uniqueness," equity versus equality, being a good friend, how to calm/self-regulate, being safe, and so on.
- Read current research on supporting racialized students and their wellness (see School Mental Health Ontario, SMHO)

CONCLUSION

Although Keshawn attended a public school with a culturally diverse student population, there were very few other families with a similar Jamaican heritage as his family. As Khalifa (2018) posits,

> Culture, it turns out, is the way that every brain makes sense of the world. That is why everyone, regardless of race or ethnicity, has a culture. Think of culture as software for the brain's hardware. The brain uses cultural information to turn everyday happenings into meaningful events. If we want to help dependent learners do more high order thinking and problem solving, then we have to access their brain's cognitive structures to deliver culturally responsive instruction. (p. 23)

It was not until his teacher(s) and administration fully embraced a socio-ecological model of support for Keshawn that infused his culture into his learning activities, resources, and physical classroom that resulted in a shift in his behavior and overall mental health. Supports for Keshawn's mother were also an important relational strategy that the school team sought out, with the assistance of the school social worker. They worked collectively to seek agencies that provided parenting coaching, regional respite and self-care opportunities for his family, subsidized extracurricular activities for Keshawn, and communal connections with other Jamaican families in the broader neighborhood. The "village" metaphor was a powerful realization for school staff to center in their work with children (Khalifa, 2018). Keshawn's case had an inspiring ripple effect within the school's collective efficacy to support other families who were traditionally labeled as at-risk. Students and families were empowered as culturally rich school partners. Staff shifted their support lens to one that nurtured "at-hope" opportunities that prioritized student wellness AND their culture.

COMMUNITY RESOURCES

- Innovative Supports for Black Parents: https://www.blackparenting.ca
- Parents of Black Children: https://parentsofblackchildren.org
- SMHO—Understanding Anti-Black Racism to Support Mental Health and Well-Being of Black and Racialized Students: https://smho-smso.ca/blog/online-resources/understanding-anti-black-racism-to-support-mental-health-and-well-being-of-black-and-racialized-students/
- Dena Simmons—Six Ways to be an Antiracist Educator: https://www.edutopia.org/video/6-ways-be-antiracist-educator

- Kids Help Phone: http://www.kidshelpphone.ca
- RiseUp: https://kidshelpphone.ca/get-info/support-for-black-youth-riseup -powered-by-kids-help-phone/
- Black Youth Helpline: https://blackyouth.ca

LINKS TO RELEVANT ONLINE MATERIALS/VIDEOS

- Student Safety Plans: https://www.ontario.ca/document/workplace-violence -school-boards-guide-law/student-safety-plan
- The Brown Bookshelf: https://thebrownbookshelf.com/2021/01/03/african -american-childrens-book-projects-best-picture-books-of-2020/
- How to Practice Culturally Responsive School Leadership—Dr. Muhammad Khalifa: https://raciallyjustschools.com/2021/09/19/how-to-practice -culturally-responsive-school-leadership/
- Khalifa's Culturally Responsive School Leadership Framework: https:// www.cehd.umn.edu/assets/docs/policy-breakfast/UMN-Culturally -Responsive-School-Leadership-Framework.pdf
- Black Child: A poem about social injustice: https://kidshelpphone.ca/get -info/black-child-a-poem-about-social-injustice
- ETFO's 365 Black Canadian Curriculum: https://members.etfo.ca/support-ingmembers/resources/pages/365.aspx
- ETFO's Anti-Oppressive Framework: https://www.etfo.ca/getmedia /67d7eb05-4c08-414a-8979-7d98d94899bc/210504_Anti-Oppressive-Booklet.pdf

REFERENCES

Bronfenbrenner, U. (1977). Toward an experimental psychology of human development. *American Psychologist, 32*(7), 515–531. https://doi.org/10.1037/0003-066X .32.7.513.

Henderson, D. X., DeCuir-Gunby, J., & Gill, V. (2016). "It *really* takes a village": A socio-ecological model of resilience for prevention among economically disadvantaged ethnic minority youth. *Journal of Primary Prevention, 37*, 469–485. https:// doi.org/10.1007/s10935-016-0446-3.

Khalifa, M. (2018). *Culturally responsive school leadership*. Harvard Education Press. https://www.crsli.org.

Chapter 2

Case Story #2—Embracing Body Diversity to Prevent Eating Disorders in a Classroom Setting in Canada

Margaret Janse van Rensburg

THEORETICAL MODEL AND BACKGROUND

The following is a case study of Morgan, age eleven in a Grade 6 classroom, who is in the early stages of an eating disorder. A Health At Every Size® (HAES® pronounced hays) informed approach is adopted by her teacher. Health At Every Size® is a movement that recognizes the inherent dignity, rights, and strengths of all people, celebrating body diversity. HAES® was developed by Lindo Bacon (formerly Linda Bacon) and Lucy Aphramor (2011), who after years of working with clients and researching nutrition, identified that purposeful food restriction (diets) can cause disordered eating, low self-esteem, and, in general, don't work. This approach acknowledges that there are wider social determinants of health, rather than the food a person eats, and the movement a person does. HAES® actively fights against "diet culture" by questioning shame around body size and honoring all foods as good food. HAES® supports mental health by fostering self-esteem in all bodies and by challenging harmful shaming and discrimination based on size, shape, weight, and food choices. The HAES® approach is considered a best practice in preventing and treating eating disorders (Schawrtz, 2012).

This approach is valuable because Morgan is in her early teens and is going through puberty. While Morgan is gaining weight, this is healthy and necessary for her development. Adopting HAES® will help her teacher navigate classroom situations which may invoke dieting desires and behaviors. Morgan's mother has shared with the school that she recently found diet pills in Morgan's knapsack. She shared that she took them away from Morgan, and Morgan is currently on a four-month waiting list to see a psychologist through a hospital in another city—the only one in the province

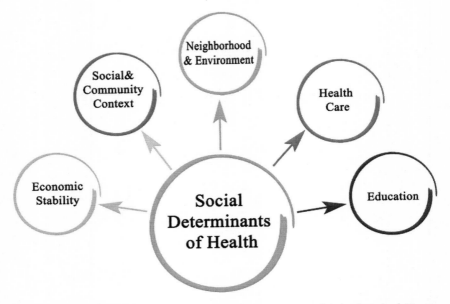

Figure 2.1 Social determinants of health. Case Story #2. *iStock—Standard License.* https://stock.adobe.com/ca/images/social-determinants-of-health/263161747?prev_url =detail.

that specializes in child eating disorders. Morgan has never had any trouble academically, having always maintained around a B-average, but has had some trouble maintaining friendships. Last year, she got into trouble for cyber-bullying another child, and within a few months was victim to bullying herself by her close friends. She has since made new friends, who she hangs out with on the cross-country running team.

MORGAN'S STORY

It's lunchtime and I'm sitting in the classroom, as my homeroom sits in the cafeteria area with the other Grade 8 classes during lunch. I get a call from a colleague who is supervising the lunchroom about an incident during lunch. Morgan had taken "anything with sugar" from the other girls' lunches in her class and thrown the food into the garbage. Morgan was overheard saying, "You'll thank me when you're not fat" to the girls as a way to justify her act. While the primary school in your neighborhood does have a "no chips, chocolate, candy, or pop" policy, the middle school is more flexible, identifying that allowing these foods encourages normal eating behaviors and moderation and that oftentimes these convenience foods may also be sent because of financial barriers to noncommercial alternatives.

I think to myself about how these thoughts about food, and the fear of fat, have led to Morgan's personal struggles with her eating. How can I demonstrate, not only to Morgan but to the other people in the class, that they do not have to fear food, fear weight gain, and they can celebrate and live happy lives in their own bodies?

I send out an email to Morgan's other teachers speaking about my concerns about weight stigma and food shame. We all commit to not speaking judgmentally about food or exercise and to treat all of the students the same, regardless of body size. We also develop a plan to deal with situations in which students make judgmental comments about food, diets, weight, shape, size, and movement. In these instances, we first question why they think that may be true? Then we propose an alternative.

On Tuesday, a student brought in mini donuts to celebrate their birthday. Morgan said, "Doughnuts aren't worth it: a moment on the lips, forever on the hips." I asked Morgan, "What makes you say that?" and Morgan replied, "It's what my sister's friend told me." I offered an alternative thought. "All foods are good foods. All bodies are good bodies." By modeling positive food talk, I am able to destigmatize food and body size in this situation,

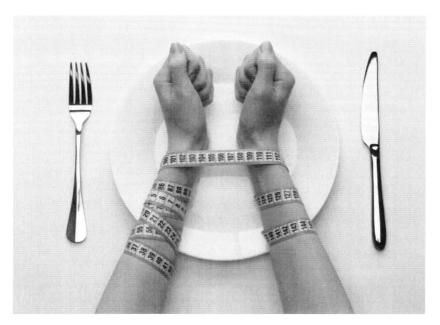

Figure 2.2   Weight stigma and food shame. Case Story #2. *iStock—Standard License.* https://stock.adobe.com/ca/images/modern-art-activity-about-anorexia-as-an-eating-disorder-characterized-by-an-abnormally-low-body-weight-cropped-shot-of-female-hands-tied-with-tape-measure-above-empty-plate-and-cutlery-on-the-table/363846575?prev_url=detail.

showing Morgan and her classmates that food is not something that needs to be restricted or policed.

BRIEF CRITICAL RESPONSE QUESTIONS

1. Have you ever found yourself educating students or friends about food or movement even though that is not the topic of your class? What kinds of beliefs do you have around food that do not promote a HAES® approach?
2. What might you do if you find diet culture in course content that you are teaching? How might you augment that information at the moment?
3. Look up HAES® social media influencers. How does the HAES® approach better prepare you to create an inclusive classroom for students with exceptionalities, students of color, and newcomer students?

REFLECTIVE RESPONSE QUESTIONS

1. Identify what you would do in response if you were the colleague who called Morgan's teacher during the first scenario. How would you respond in a HAES® informed way to Morgan throwing out other students' food?
2. What barriers do you think that Morgan's teacher faced in getting their colleagues to adopt a HAES® informed attitude?
3. Morgan's mother calls you. She says she is worried that Morgan has not been eating her lunch. What strategies could you apply in ensuring that Morgan is eating her lunch while respecting your own boundaries and your relationship with Morgan?
4. Morgan has left for residential treatment for an eating disorder in Toronto. How do you inform the other students of Morgan leaving? Create a plan to stop any gossip that may result.
5. Do you think that there could be many times that a HAES® informed approach is not appropriate? Investigate online resources to justify your answer.

Strategies of Support to Consider

- When offering physical education and movement in class, thinking about adapting the movements so that they are accessible to all children.
- Do not weigh children or line them up by size (even height!) This evaluation of body size can be harmful. Avoid associating movement with health and rather present it as an enjoyable activity for children.
- Have diverse visitors to the classroom to model that success is not based being in a white, cisnormative, and thin body.

- Track your own thoughts, feelings, and actions that are not in line with HAES® principles using a Thought Record (e.g., sample thought record in Appendix B).
- Create moments to make sure that all students feel successful in class that is external to body size and shape or food behaviors.
- Avoid assignments, classes, or assigning books that center on types of eating disorders and behaviors. This increases stigmatization and may model behaviors for students to adopt.
- Show movies on body and size diversity.
  - Strong! A documentary by Julie Wyman that follows the story of Cheryl Haworth and her journey as a weight lifter.
- Post posters around school that feature persons of diversity.
  - Stand4Kids posters, an initiative by Marilyn Wann, include photos of diverse individuals with captions promoting self-love, self-acceptance, and dismantling fatphobia and diet culture.
- Use the Everybody in Schools Curriculum Unit Resource Kit to assess your school and teach the following curriculum:
  - Self-esteem and resilience
  - Active living
  - Healthy and pleasurable eating
  - Valuing body size diversity

CONCLUSION

Promoting health through dieting and food restriction is associated with the development of eating disorders and is a predictor of weight gain in adolescence (Fothergill et al., 2016; Newmark-Sztainer et al., 2007). Overall, dieting has been demonstrated as ineffective for the majority of people (McEvedy et al., 2017; Patton et al., 1999). Therefore, it is important to adopt a HAES® weight-inclusive approach. In adopting this approach, it is important to reflect on your own biases and beliefs surrounding weight and consider how these biases and beliefs may impact the diverse children whom you work with. Operant learning theory identifies that behaviors increase in certain settings if reinforced, and decrease if they are not (Skinner, 1938). Further, social learning theory theorizes that people learn from one another through observation, imitation, and modeling (Bandura, 1971). Therefore, by modeling HAES® in your classroom, setting up environments where all bodies are celebrated, and reinforcing behaviors that are body inclusive, teachers can assist in reducing stigma and bullying surrounding body diversity.

Sometimes parents, caregivers, other teachers may be on diets, and children in classes may also be on special diets. This is OK, and it is not your responsibility to change everyone's thoughts and behavior. In these instances, teachers have the responsibility to protect the children in their classroom from food and weight stigma (see Appendix A). In cases where a student is identified with an eating disorder, there may be ongoing collaboration necessary with registered dietitians, psychologists, psychiatrists, social workers, hospitals, and family. In these instances, it is important to value the perspective of the parent in assisting with the health and well-being of the child, while respecting the privacy of the child. In adopting a HAES® approach, teachers assist children in preventing eating disorders.

LINKS TO RELEVANT RESOURCES

- Association for Size Diversity and Health. The HAES® Approach. https://www.sizediversityandhealth.org/content.asp?id=76
- Association for Size Diversity and Health. Resources. https://www.sizediversityandhealth.org/content.asp?id=35&category=Children%2FTeens
- Bacon, L. Resources for Parents/Teachers/School Administrators. https://lindobacon.com/_resources/resources-for-teachersadministrators/
- Food Psych Podcast with Christy Harrison. https://christyharrison.com/foodpsych
- Government of Canada. (2019). The Social Determinants of Health. https://www.canada.ca/en/public-health/services/health-promotion/population-health/what-determines-health.html
- Health At Every Size® Registry of professionals https://haescommunity.com/search/
- Stand4Kids. (2012). Posters. https://fatkidsunited.wordpress.com/2012/01/23/stand4kids-tumblr/#more-71
- Strong! A film by Julie Wyman. http://strongthefilm.com/
- The National Association to Advance Fat Acceptance. Everybody in Schools HAES Toolkit. https://www.naafaonline.com/dev2/education/haesschool.html
- The National Association to Advance Fat Acceptance. Child Advocacy Tool Kit. https://www.naafaonline.com/dev2/about/Brochures/NAAFA_Child_Advocacy_Toolkit.pdf

BOOKS

Bacon, L. (2010). *Health at every size* (2nd ed.). Ben Bella Books.
Bacon, L., & Apramor, L. (2014). *Body respect: What conventional health books get wrong, leave out, and just plain fail to understand about weight.* Benbella Books.

Harrison, C. (2019). *Anti-diet: Reclaim your time, money, well-being, and happiness through eating*. Little Brown Spark.

Wolf, N. (2009). *The beauty myth: How images of beauty are used against women*. Harper Collins.

REFERENCES

Bacon, L., & Aphramor, L. (2011). Weight science: Evaluating the evidence for a paradigm shift. *BioMed Central Nutrition Journal*, *10*(9). https://doi.org/10.1186/1475-2891-10-9.

Bandura, A. (1971). *Social learning theory*. http://www.asecib.ase.ro/mps/Bandura_SocialLearningTheory.pdf.

Fothergill, E., Guo, J., Howard, L., Kerns, J., Knuth, N., Brychta, R., Chen, K., Skarulis, M., Walter, M., Walter, P., & Hall, K. (2016). Persistent metabolic adaptation 6 years after "The Biggest Loser" competition. *Obesity*, *24*(8), 1612–1619. https://doi.org/10.1002/oby.21538.

McEvedy, S. M., Sullivan-Mort, G., McLean, S. A., Pascoe, M. C., & Paxton, S. J. (2017). Ineffectiveness of commercial weight-loss programs for achieving modest but meaningful weight loss: Systematic review and meta-analysis. *Journal of Health Psychology*. Advance online publication. https://doi.org/10.1177/1359105317705983.

Newmark-Sztainer, D., Wall, M., Haines, J., Story, M., & Eisenberg, M. (2007). Why does dieting predict weight gain in adolescents? Findings from project EAT-II: A 5-year longitudinal study. *Journal of the American Dietetic Association*, *107*(3), 448–455. https://doi.org/10.1016/j.jada.2006.12.013.

Patton, G. C., Selzer, R., Coffey, C., Carlin, J. B., & Wolfe, R. (1999). Onset of adolescent eating disorders: Population based cohort study over 3 years. *British Medical Journal*, *318*(7186), 765–768. https://doi.org/10.1136/bmj.318.7186.765.

Schawrtz, D. (2012). *What is health at every size*. National Eating Disorders Association. https://pdfs.semanticscholar.org/30cf/cb3df0dfc20cda736d395b1e4af9ed2fd52a.pdf.

Skinner, B. F. (1938). *The behavior of organisms: An experimental analysis*. Appleton-Century.

APPENDIX A

Sample phrases to challenge body shame and food shame
Creating a safer space
- ◦ We don't judge food in this space.
- ◦ We don't talk about bodies in that way here.

- Let's avoid speaking about the value of foods in the classroom.
- Let's change the topic to anything but food/weight/shape.

Challenging fat stigma and modeling size acceptance
- All bodies are good bodies.
- People are not fat, they have fat.
- It's not fun to think about weight, there are so many other interesting things to think about.
- People can be healthy and happy no matter their size/shape/weight.

Challenging diet talk and modeling healthy eating
- Life is easier when we don't have to worry about what we eat.
- Some people eat special foods because their bodies need it, it's good to try lots of different foods to see what your body likes and doesn't like.
- There are no good or bad foods, just foods that some people like and that others don't.
- Food is a great way of bringing people together.

APPENDIX B

Thought Record (example)
Where were you:
At the gym, on the treadmill
Emotion/Feeling:
Guilt
Automatic Thought:
I need to burn off calories from pizza lunch
Evidence that supports this thought:
Pizza is a calorie-dense food
Evidence that does not support this thought:
Pizza has all food groups and satisfies me
Eating pizza in moderation prevents me from overeating
Everyone deserves food for lunch
My body will digest calories from all food I eat
Impact of automatic thought on behavior with students:

> I might tell a student that pizza is not a good food, even if their parents do not have resources to feed them something alternative
> I may shame students for eating pizza on pizza day
> I may implicate that food must be burned off through exercise to students, setting an unhealthy example

Alternative thought:

> "I'm engaging in movement to make my body and mind feel good"
>
> "I'm engaging in movement because I like getting in the running-zone"

Impact of alternative thought on behavior with students:

> I am more open to accepting diverse bodies and abilities in my classroom
>
> I am able to think about the foods that my students eat as a product larger structures (food availability, cultural choices, enjoyment) rather than judge the food for societal assumptions
>
> I am better able to model healthy relationships with movement to students

Thought Record (blank)

Where were you:

    _____

    _____

    _____

Emotion/Feeling:

    _____

    _____

    _____

Automatic Thought:

    _____

    _____

    _____

Evidence that supports this thought:

    _____

    _____

    _____

Evidence that does not support this thought:

_____

_____

_____

Impact of automatic thought on behavior with students:

_____

_____

_____

Alternative thought:

_____

_____

_____

Impact of alternative thought on behavior with students:

_____

_____

_____

Chapter 3

Case Story #3—Autism and Anxiety in a Primary School-Aged Child in France

Mélissa Villella and Hélène Abdelnour

INTRODUCTION

Recent studies have shown that some students with autism spectrum disorder (ASD) also experience symptoms of anxiety; consequently, they have a unique set of mental health and well-being needs (Boulter et al., 2014; Stuart et al., 2020). In this chapter, we will examine the case of a primary school-aged child with ASD and anxiety from a mental health and well-being perspective. More specifically, this is a case study about Zoe, a five-year-old girl from Nice, France, who is entering the *Cours préparatoire* (CP) level, which is equivalent to the first year of mainstream primary or elementary school in Ontario.

To understand the complexity of this case study, a description of the family and school's pre-relationship narratives is necessary. The goal is to show that building a trusting relationship does not automatically start out that way, despite the good intentions of everyone involved. As exemplified in Zoe's case, this relationship requires a great deal of consistent and concerted work for Zoe to succeed academically and to ensure her mental health and well-being. However, this work mostly requires combined effort and communication from both the parents and school personnel.

Further explained in Zoe's narrative is the special importance of a family-school team coming together in the case of a child with ASD and anxiety. It is possible for the family-school team to build upon a common understanding of certain concepts and models in order to work together in Zoe's best interests. Also included are brief descriptions of the strategies that Mme C., Zoe's mother, and Mme L., Zoe's school principal, have chosen to help Zoe succeed in the context of France's limited in-school mental health services and support. To this end, it is important to note that in Nice, France, most specialized services outside of public institutions are paid for by parents and partially subsidized by the *Maison des Personnes Handicapées* (*MDHP*), a state-run organization for handicapped persons. However, these services are offered outside of the school context. In sum, the school and outside services, such as the ones Zoe receives, work together in a very limited fashion. The communication and relationship between the school and outside services are mostly limited to a once-a-year meeting with the *Équipe de suivi de scolarité* (*ESS*), which is the equivalent of an Identification, Placement, Revision Committee (IPRC) meeting in Ontario, Canada's schooling context, for example.

ABOUT ZOE

Zoe started school at three and a half years of age in what we call in France *la maternelle*, a three-year mainstream program, sometimes known elsewhere as kindergarten. During her first year of school, Zoe did not receive personalized support services since her ASD had not been diagnosed at that point, and she was attending school only two hours a day. During that first year, her parents opened a case with the *MDPH* in order to obtain an *Accompagnant des élèves en situation de handicap* (*AESH*), that is, a shadow teacher to accompany her during her school hours.

Unlike her peers, Zoe still did not attend school full time in her second year of *maternelle*. She attended only part time since she was allotted an *AESH* for a total of only three hours per day. However, the number of hours allotted for her to attend school increased in the third and last year of *maternelle* to a total of twenty hours. The total number of hours allotted was finally enough to enable Zoe to attend school full time since she had also started applied behavioral analysis (ABA) and speech therapy. In short, she needed the extra time for those therapies.

During the last two years of *maternelle*, the *AESH* remained the same and had learned how to help Zoe cope with her learning difficulties as well as her anxiety. To this end, it is important to keep in mind that Zoe does not have an intellectual delay. This was confirmed through testing done at the *Centre Ressource Autisme* (*CRA*) in her region, that is, an Autism Resource Centre. While Zoe's needs are more behavioral and sensory than intellectual, the school had difficulty meeting her needs due to a lack of knowledge about autism and how to adapt academic content accordingly.

In terms of special needs, Zoe has difficulty understanding abstract concepts, transitioning from one activity to the next, concentrating on a task long enough without having stereotypy, such as delayed echolalia (repeating aloud dialogues heard on TV), getting in the way of her thought process. Added to this, most children with ASD have an abnormal response to rewards and have a different reaction during feedback learning (Lin et al., 2012). Therefore, some children with ASD need more motivation and more reinforcement to keep on going than typical children (Schuetze et al., 2017). More specifically, they can be motivated by using different categories of reinforcers such as an activity that they enjoy, a tangible item such as a toy or the encouragement of both their teacher and peers; each child has his or her own preferences that can be tested for (Cooper, 2014).

Zoe also needs to overcome her difficulties in social activities such as chatting with her peers and her sensory issues such as sensitivity to noise and bright light that can create an increase in her anxiety level. Her anxiety usually manifests itself through nail and cuticle biting until bleeding occurs, increased speech volume, screaming and biting her hand every time someone says "no" to her, difficulty falling asleep, waking up in the middle of the night, and staying awake talking to herself for two to three hours at a time. In sum, these are the very behaviors that Zoe's parents and her teachers have learned to avoid triggering or to manage, both at home and at school.

That said, after three years of *maternelle*, it was time for Zoe to change schools. She would now be entering *l'écoleprimaire*, which is equivalent to primary or elementary school in some countries. However, the *AESH* announced to both the parents and the administration that she did not wish to follow Zoe to the new school. Therefore, Zoe was going to have a new *AESH* by her side whom she did not know. This made Zoe's parents somewhat nervous given all the time and work it had taken to organize adequate in-school services for Zoe up to that point and the fact that all these changes might trigger an increase in Zoe's anxiety and lead to problem behaviors in school.

During the summer break, which is usually all of July and August, Zoe's family also moved to a new house in a different neighborhood. Luckily for all, the schools in the new neighborhood had a great reputation for being accepting and keeping a close eye on the children. However, once again, Zoe would need to make new friends, and most of all, other students would need to get to know her and accept her with her differences. In short, Zoe was facing many uncertainties: a new neighborhood, a new house, a new school, a new *AESH*, and new friends. This is important to note since some children with ASD have difficulties coping effectively with uncertainty, and this situation was going to be a real challenge (Pellicano & Burr, 2012). As such, coping with change may create a great deal of anxiety for children, such as Zoe.

Nevertheless, Zoe had always surprised everyone with her ability to "keep on swimming" like Dory from the Disney movie *Trouver Nemo* (*Finding Nemo*) (Disney, 2003). More specifically, Zoe was navigating an ocean of knowledge and a world that could sometimes be hostile to her. During the first two years of a three-year *maternelle/* kindergarten program, however, the

AESH had managed to get her to work. The more the *AESH* came to know her, the more she was able to put strategies in place to reduce Zoe's anxiety and draw the best out of her. The relationship between the *AESH*, her parents, the professionals surrounding Zoe, and the school personnel had been such that the child had been able to advance academically, socially, and in her overall behavior.

Now, however, it was time for Zoe to attend primary school and for a new support system to be put in place to enable her to succeed and overcome her anxiety. Her parents would, therefore, have to build bridges with the new school's principal, for example, in order to facilitate Zoe's adaptation and make sure that this new environment did not exacerbate her anxiety.

The following narratives, that is, Mme C., Zoe's mother, and Mme L., the school principal, first describe what a new pre-relationship narrative for both the family and the school may look like. These two narratives are included so that the reader can better understand a mother's perspective, as well as a school principal's when a family-school team has not yet been established. We have also included Zoe's voice in her own narrative, which will be presented at the end of the case study. The goal here is to give the final word to Zoe, a five-year-old child with ASD and anxiety, since her success and well-being should ideally serve as a gentle reminder that her needs must remain at the center of the family-school relationship. That said, it is time to discover Zoe's mother's narrative.

MME C.: MOTHER'S PRE-RELATIONSHIP STORY

Below you will read Zoe's mother's narrative before her first meeting with the principal of her child's new school.

What can we expect this time? Will they understand her needs and agree to put in place what she needs to help her advance? I know it's work. Hard work. I know they have many students that they need to attend to, and my daughter isn't the easiest one. But she is worth it. She has progressed so much. If only they could have seen her at age three. She was so different, and she has changed completely thanks to being in mainstream school imitating her peers and thanks to her therapy.

As I walk to my meeting with the principal of the new school, our life of the past few years is flashing before my eyes: "Your daughter is depressed because you love her too much"; "No, your daughter is not autistic. Why do you want to put a label on her?"; "She has autism; she should be in the class for handicapped children where all people with autism belong"; "She is not able to understand the math problems, she's not up to the level of her class"; "I love working with your daughter, I have learned so much especially about different ways of teaching the same thing"; "Your daughter has changed me forever and I am thankful that I have had her in my class"; "Your daughter is full of surprises."

Every year, with the help of time management strategies, antecedent strategies and relaxation techniques, we were able to get her to overcome her difficulties, such as anxiety, and to support her in continuing to advance at school.

How will it be this time? This new school . . . Will I have to wait for months again before they agree to put in place the same strategies that we have already tested at home? These strategies work, I swear, and will make their lives easier. But why, every year, do they wait so long before they agree to talk to me, to listen? I know I am her mother, so, of course, I think she's a great kid. But I have realistic expectations for her. I trained hard to learn the discipline that has been helping her blossom, by earning a master's degree and becoming certified in ABA. I can help if they would only let me. I hope they will listen so that we can work as a team. Zoe deserves it. She has been working so hard just to be able to stay where she belongs. My heart is pounding as I open the door to the meeting room.

As can be seen, Zoe's mother not only has firsthand experience with her child but also professional knowledge about her daughter's diagnosis and the treatment strategies that have been helping her. And mostly, she wishes to adopt a preventive approach with the school to ensure that her daughter's best interests are met.

In the meantime, the school principal also has a personal narrative going on before this meeting. Now, let's explore that one too.

MME L.: SCHOOL PRINCIPAL'S PRE-RELATIONSHIP STORY

Below is the narrative of the school principal regarding Zoe's mother's preventive approach, that is, calling a school meeting before the academic year has even started.

I have been given a heads-up by the previous school principal, whom I barely know, that these parents are really "involved," especially the mother. In fact, it is early May, and I have already received a request for a team meeting way before the end of the year. The mother also indicated that the first meeting could happen at the very latest during the week before school starts with myself, the classroom teacher, as well as the AESH and various specialists. The mother has also asked me to share my special education philosophy with her, especially how it pertains to school children with ASD and anxiety management. She also wants to know what my knowledge of ASD, ABA and anxiety are. The icing on the cake was when she asked me if I knew what percentage of girls have been diagnosed with ASD and anxiety, and what a school transition might look like, based on my previous experience.

Now, I am all for welcoming new parents and students to the school in order to ease the family's and the student's new school jitters. So, I have decided to do this first meeting by myself in July since everyone is already on vacation. However, I simply could not schedule anything earlier because of the current school year's challenges, such as school starting and stopping due to Covid-19. Also, my staff assignments have yet to be finished, and I am still hiring for her daughter's class. So, I already know that I cannot give the mother all the answers that she may want from the get-go. Will this meeting, which will be short on answers, stress her out more, or will this discussion be our first building blocks toward a long-term fruitful partnership? Anyway, here we go . . . before the rest of my meetings today. Ouf! [Argh!]

The secretary has just buzzed me to tell me the mother is on the way to my door. (Knock, knock) Bonjour, Mme C., please come into my office, how are you doing today?

As can be seen, the school principal demonstrated a certain willingness to meet the mother and did so before the end of the school year. However, the school principal was not able to meet with her as early as the mother would have liked for various reasons. This gap might have caused some tension from the outset.

Through these two short narratives, we hope that families and/or school personnel reading them may develop a better understanding of the pre-relationship narratives of both Mme C., the mother, and Mme L., the school principal, and how they can impact new family-school relationships. The beginning of any new family-school relationship is never an easy one for either parents or school principals. Both have their own areas of expertise, knowledge, and priorities. Yet, both parties needed to learn to work together in a timely fashion for the success, health, and well-being of Zoe, a child with both ASD and anxiety.

IMPORTANCE OF FAMILY-SCHOOL RELATIONSHIPS

With regard to the importance of building a solid family-school team relationship, some would argue that this is crucial for every child's success and well-being. However, for two specific reasons, this particular relationship is even more important for the long-term success and well-being of a student with ASD who also has anxiety. First, the behaviors of a child with ASD and anxiety are not only more complex than many other students' needs, but these behaviors may also change in more significant ways over time (Stuart et al., 2020). For example, a child with ASD and anxiety may experience extreme obsessional avoidance behaviors in relation to everyday life demands as of a young age (Stuart et al., 2020; O'Nions et al., 2014). Second, they may also develop less tolerance for uncertainty in their everyday lives during adolescence even though their extreme obsessional avoidance behaviors may decrease (Buhr & Dugas, 2009; Stuart et al., 2020). In fact, according to Stuart et al. (2020),

> one possible explanation is that with increasing age comes the development of new strategies that may be less demand avoidant for managing IU, such that EDA behaviour becomes less explicit. Alternatively, those placing demands on the child, such as parents and teachers, may have learned over time to avoid or disguise demands to avoid extreme reactions. (p. 65)

In other words, according to these authors, it is important for the family-school team to understand the relationship between extreme demand avoidance (EDA) and intolerance of uncertainty (IU) in order to contribute favorably to the mental health of a child with ASD and anxiety. As such, a parent like Mme C. and a school principal like Mme L. may turn to empirical-based research models and theories for some guidance on how to help children with ASD who also experience anxiety.

THEORETICAL MODEL AND BACKGROUND

Having a common understanding of theoretical concepts and models may be important to families and school personnel alike. In general, Gingras and Côté (2016) explain that "to avoid misunderstandings, any theory must define its concepts precisely" (unofficial translation, p. 108). As such, there must be a common understanding of the concepts of ASD, ABA, and anxiety in order to fully comprehend Zoe's narrative. There must also be a brief presentation of the theoretical frameworks that are complementary to both concepts from a mental health and wellness perspective. The overall goal is to ground the case study in evidence-based practices (EBP) that align with ABA favorable to children with ASD (Slocum et al., 2014). It is also to apply these EBPs to a theoretical model of IU that takes into account how anxiety manifests itself in children and adolescents with ASD (Boulter et al., 2014). That said, it is time to discuss the definition and criteria of ASD.

AUTISM SPECTRUM DISORDER (ASD)

Healthcare professionals use the fifth version of the American Psychiatric Association's *Diagnostic and Statistical Manual (DSM-5)* to classify and diagnose a variety of disorders, including such neurodevelopmental disorders as ASD. However, some professionals, including psychologists, may also use other tools to evaluate for ASD (Kulage et al., 2020), for example, the Autism Diagnosis Observation Schedule (ADOS) (Lord et al., 2012).

While ASD has been included as a unique disorder since the inception of the third version (i.e., DSM-3), the definition and criteria have undergone some important changes in the fifth version of the guide. Today, there is a newer overarching category that is known as ASD rather than the former subcategories of Asperger syndrome, pervasive developmental disorder (nonspecific), and autism. As Tsai (2012) explains, "This change reflects the thought that the symptoms of these subtypes represent a continuum from mild to severe, rather than being distinct disorders" (p. 1011). Therefore, medical professionals generally no longer refer, for example, to Asperger syndrome as distinct from a nonspecific pervasive developmental disorder, as was the case in the past (Tsai, 2012).

APPLIED BEHAVIORAL ANALYSIS (ABA)

ABA is a science-based discipline used to study and modify behavior for the purpose of improving socially significant behaviors. On the one hand, ABA uses individualized procedures to reduce behaviors that manifest themselves in excess and, on the other hand, to increase behaviors that are absent or present at too low a level (Abdelnour, 2019).

In fact, environmental variables, which have a functional relationship with the target behaviors, are discovered and then manipulated to shape the behaviors of interest (Cooper et al., 2014).

In addition, ABA is mainly recognized in France as the treatment of choice for ASD and has been recommended by the *HAS (Haute Autorité de Santé)*, which is equivalent to Ontario Autism Program in Ontario, Canada. It is also unique in the fact that the treatment is applied in all the natural environments of the child, such as the home, school, extracurricular activities, and so on. Most of the time, therapists either provoke behavior in order to be able to apply the treatment selected or they simply take advantage of a spontaneous occurrence of behavior in the natural environment to execute the treatment selected (Bailey & Burch, 2016). In sum, ABA focuses on behavior, not on a diagnosis or hypothetical reasons for the occurrence of the behavior. For example, it does not concentrate on the ASD label but instead aims to modify behavioral excesses and deficits that are present in a person living with ASD (Cooper et al., 2014).

EVIDENCE-BASED PRACTICE (EBP)

The first framework relates to ASD. More precisely, we will be referring to EBP framework since this particular EBP model aligns with ABA and is used with certain clients, such as children with ASD. According to Slocum et al. (2014), an EBP model is best described as "a decision-making process that integrates: (a) the best available evidence with; (b) clinical expertise; and © client values and context" (p. 44). In other words, it is not only perceived by some researchers as a whole person approach but it is also seen as a whole family approach.

Their EBP model has some unique advantages. It uses the best available evidence, based on both scientific and professional knowledge, when deciding on human-resource allocations and initiatives (Slocum et al., 2014). It is also based on empirically sound short-term and long-term treatment for the good of both the client and society. Second, as for practitioners' clinical expertise, this can be summed up as follows: (a) knowing current research literature and how to apply it with particular clients; (b) incorporating ABA and using expertise in applying clinical and interpersonal skill sets; (c) integrating client values and taking into consideration the context; (d) recognizing the necessity for outside consultations; and (e) decision-making based on data and continued professional development (Slocum et al., 2014). Finally, Slocum et al. (2014) insist that the social validity of this model is an integral part of contextual appropriateness as it pertains to the individuals who not only implement treatments but also manage other environmental aspects of treatment implementation.

Given that this case study is focused on Zoe, a five-year-old student with ASD and anxiety who receives ABA and has been attending mainstream school in France, this particular theoretical framework is a foundational way of perceiving the family and the school as equal and important partners in their interactions when dealing with a child with ASD.

We now need to turn to a discussion of Zoe's anxiety.

ANXIETY

In this case study, it is important to note that we are referring to anxiety and not to an anxiety disorder per se. According to Pilkington et al. (2007), the difference between the two concepts can be described as follows:

> Anxiety has been defined as a "persistent feeling of dread, apprehension and impending disaster or tension and uneasiness." The term "anxiety disorders" is used as an umbrella term for a number of conditions including panic

disorder, phobias, obsessive-compulsive disorder, generalized anxiety, trau-
matic stress disorder and anxiety disorder due to a general medical condition.
(p. 152)

In other words, feeling anxious does not equate to having an anxiety disorder that has been diagnosed via a health professional using the DSM-5 or
other diagnostic tools.

Given the important distinction that we have briefly defined and what is
included/excluded in the definition of anxiety, we can now examine a complementary model of intolerance of uncertainty of anxiety (IC) by Boulter
et al. (2014) in relation to this case study.

INTOLERANCE OF UNCERTAINTY (IU) FOR ANXIETY

In order to better understand the IU in children and adolescents with ASD,
one should understand not only the underlying factors but also the manifested
behaviors. In particular, such a model by Boutler et al. (2014) is useful. On
the one hand, these authors explain that three factors contribute to an IU: (1)
social/environmental factors; (2) rigidity of thought and difficulty with emotional processing; and (3) sensory sensitivities. On the other hand, the factors
that create IU lead to two behaviors: (1) restricted and repetitive behaviors
(RRB) and (2) anxiety. According to Wigham et al. (2015), who studied the
relationships between sensory processing, repetitive behaviors and the potential role of IU and anxiety among youth with ASD:

> Restricted and repetitive behaviours are core features of ASD. RRBs encompass
> behaviours and preoccupations which are characteristically restricted and inflex-
> ible, such as repetitive language or movements, insistence on the same routines,
> and circumscribed interests. (p. 945)

In other words, we should not dissociate RRBs from ASD and anxiety.

In this conceptual framework section, a common understanding of the
foundational theoretical frameworks that guide Zoe's family-school relationship has been established. We will now identify and explain a few basic strategies that both Zoe's parents and her school's staff can apply at home and at
school, respectively, to best meet her needs.

STRATEGIES

Given that Zoe's academic success and her mental health and well-being are
equally important, we will propose some basic—but specific—instructional

accommodations, environmental accommodations, and assessment accommodations. In fact, the parents and school personnel alike can use these accommodations at home and at school, respectively. The goal here is to streamline Zoe's use of these strategies between home and school so that she can generalize their usage while ensuring that the family-school team remains on the same page.

ESTABLISHING COMMUNICATION

While there are many ways to establish an open and effective communication relationship between the parents and school personnel, we will concentrate on suggesting three ways of doing so in the context of this case study. The three ways are as follows: (1) implementing a *cahier de liaison*, that is, a family-school communication book; (2) establishing monthly meetings in order to check in together on Zoe's progress and adapt her material; (3) having the ABA supervisor and the therapist in charge of establishing her programs regularly visit/observe Zoe in school so that they can better adapt the strategies which the family, the school, and the *AESH* need to put in place.

ANTECEDENT STRATEGIES

In ABA, we analyze behavior as being part of a three-term contingency known as antecedent behavior consequences (ABC). According to Skinner (2014), every behavior has an "antecedent," which is what happens right before a given behavior. Then, there is the "behavior" itself which Skinner (2014) describes in specific, measurable, and observable terms. Following the "behavior," there are the "consequences" of this behavior. In other words, we must ask ourselves: Was the behavior in question reinforced? Punished? The answer will help us determine the probability of such behavior happening again in the future.

Antecedent strategies are strategies put in place before the occurrence of the behavior in order to reduce or entirely eliminate the probability of the occurrence of a behavior. For example, a child with ASD always starts screaming when entering a specific room. Following an assessment of the function of this child's behavior, it was discovered that the flickering of the bright lights was unbearable because of his sensory issues. In order to stop the screaming, we can repair the light and make sure it is dimmed to a comfortable level before asking the child to enter. The probability of a child with ASD entering the room without screaming will be higher now that we have modified the environment and removed the aversive factor before the behavior of screaming occurred (Cooper et al., 2014).

In sum, antecedent strategies can be suggested at home and at school. However, they are especially important at school since we do not want children with ASD to have disruptive behaviors that may lead them to being labeled as bad by their peers or even expelled from school. Below are a few strategies that can be used.

TIME MANAGEMENT

Children with ASD and anxiety often have rigidities and executive functions deficits that lead to difficulties in transitions between two activities (Boutler et al., 2014). They need help with transitioning because such change creates a great deal of anxiety that manifests through problem behaviors such as a refusal to let go of what they were doing or starting a new activity, and behavioral problems such as screaming and avoiding the work they are supposed to do (Cihak et al., 2010; Cohen & Volkmar, 1997).

In order to ease this anxiety of the unknown, several strategies can be put in place, such as the use of a Time Timer (https://www.timetimer.com/), a simple clock that shows the remaining time in red. Now that the time left can be clearly seen, the child may be able to complete the activity without difficulty.

Another strategy is the use of a visual activity schedule/agenda, which is considered a visual prompt. The different activities that need to be completed are presented to a child with ASD and anxiety in a visual form, such as pictograms depicting each activity to be done in the allotted time. For example, we could have one image for *math*, followed by an image for *drawing*; and this would be followed by an image for *recess*, another for *French*, an image for *reading*, and one for *going home*. Once the activity is completed, the corresponding image is removed. This particular strategy has been shown to be efficient in enabling some children with ASD and anxiety to comprehend what is expected of them, and particularly what is coming next. It eases the anxiety of the unknown since the time lapse is now organized and planned for. Furthermore, the child can see his or her next break, and this can be a motivation to finish the work (Heflin & Simpson, 1998; Knight et al., 2014).

It is important to note that these and any other strategies should be individualized to each child's ability and comprehension. In middle school, for instance, the agenda could be written instead of visual and show the full day. These techniques can be used in school as well as in the family environment to plan the week and especially trips or outings because, as added activities, such excursions tend to exacerbate anxiety.

ADJUSTING THE LEVEL OF DIFFICULTY

Another strategy that can be used is adapting the level of difficulty of an exercise and the level of guidance to a child's ability. For example, we can provide children with ASD and anxiety with a lot of guidance by helping them physically or by giving them step-by-step help to accomplish what is asked. If a child needs to write the letter "Z," for example, we can place our hand over the child's hand and draw the letter together. As he or she becomes more proficient, we can gradually withdraw our guidance by first placing our hand on the child's wrist and then on the elbow and finally discontinuing our help entirely.

In addition, visual guidance could be put in place, such as little dots that a young child with ASD and anxiety will need to follow in order to trace a letter. The dots can be very close to one other at the beginning and, as the child learns to trace the letter, we can space them out gradually so that they eventually form only the end points of the letter. And then we remove the guiding dots entirely.

In the case of an exercise that requires several steps to arrive at a conclusion, such as "I buy 2 pieces of fruit for 2 euros each and I give a 10 euro bill to the cashier. How much will she give me back?," we can help a child with ASD and anxiety by drawing the fruit on a sheet of paper to eliminate the abstract aspect of the exercise or by indicating the steps to follow in a checklist. For example, (1) How many pieces of fruit are you buying?; (2) Draw the fruit; (3) How much is each piece of fruit?; (4) How much should you pay for the two pieces of fruit? Do the calculation; (5) How much did you give the cashier?; (6) What are we looking for? What is the appropriate mathematical operation (+, −, ×, /) to use?; (7) Perform the operation and; (8) Write down the result.

This strategy reduces anxiety by showing children what is required of them together with the steps that will lead them to the desired result. In sum, we have removed the uncertainty factor (Boutler et al., 2014). This also has the advantage of promoting autonomy because it involves reliance on the child's checklist rather than on another person to complete the exercise.

Finally, the level of difficulty can also be adjusted by reducing the number of items that a child with ASD and anxiety needs to complete. For example, in a math exercise, instead of five calculations, the child could be asked to complete only two. The demand we are placing on the child can increase gradually as he or she manages to accomplish what is being asked. Moreover, in the family environment, this guidance can be given during the morning routine: physical guidance for brushing teeth, for example, visual guidance for the steps involved in properly showering, and so on.

SPACE MANAGEMENT

Another useful strategy is the management of the space in which children with ASD and anxiety are working. To avoid distractions, these children should be seated close to the board and near the teacher. Such a strategy will help avoid visual distractions when other children are moving about the classroom and will reduce extraneous noises interfering with the teacher's instruction. It will allow children with ASD and anxiety to concentrate better and avoid becoming anxious because of what is going on around them in the classroom. We need to remember that something that may be very bearable to us, such as another child playing with a pen, can overstimulate a child with ASD and create a peak in anxiety and distraction because it mobilizes all of this child's cognitive resources.

Another strategy along the same lines of space management would be clear the table of everything except the tools required for the actual work. Again, this will remove unnecessary distractions. In a family environment, the same techniques can also be used for homework.

RELAXATION TECHNIQUES

Reducing the anxiety experienced in the school environment by children with ASD improves their overall school functioning as well as their long-term outcomes in life (Hillman et al., 2020). Following the implementation of the first line of antecedent intervention strategies, anxiety management can be proposed in order to break the chain of stimuli that lead to anxiety and redirect the nervous system to a state of calm (Lynch, 2019).

Diaphragmatic breathing, commonly called "belly" breathing since this is where the breathing occurs, can be used to increase the oxygen taken in and promote slower deeper breathing. For example, children with ASD and anxiety can place their hands on their stomachs and try "belly" breathing as they raise and lower their hands at least five times.

Another physical technique is progressive muscle relaxation (PMR) (Lynch, 2019). When arousal of anxiety occurs, the person is unaware of the muscle tensions that he or she is experiencing. In this method, each muscle group is tensed strongly before it is released. For example, we can ask a child with ASD and anxiety to squeeze his or her hands together for three seconds and then release them. We next move to the arms and then the shoulders and so on. At home, the whole body can be scanned and worked on while only the upper body can be stimulated in a school setting where the child is seated. Finally, other relaxation techniques that involve mindfulness meditation and visualization will require many adaptations, such as visual supports for children with ASD; abstract terms and metaphors should be avoided with these children because of their difficulties in comprehending them (Lynch, 2019).

In France, many of these techniques are first put in place by the therapist/ psychologist, who then trains the parents on how to do so. When the school applies the same techniques, this helps a child with ASD and anxiety to generalize them and reinforce their natural use and efficiency.

REINFORCEMENT

We should not forget that, throughout all of the strategies proposed, the child needs to know clearly what is expected of him or her. Therefore, we need to use simple words or images. More importantly still, once the target behavior is reached, it should be reinforced in a number of ways: socially ("Well done! You did a great job reading!"); tangibly ("You can now play with your toy for three minutes while the other children are finishing their work."); and/or by letting the child escape all the demands and have a break in which to do as he or she pleases. It is very important to reinforce the appropriate behavior and to increase the probability of the child's engaging in the desirable behavior again.

CONCLUSION

In this brief case study, we have included the perspectives of a family-school team to demonstrate the complexity of this relationship and indicate the actions the team can take to effectively collaborate and support a child with ASD and anxiety. More specifically, we have been privy to a mother's narrative and a school principal's pre-relationship narrative as they pertain to Zoe, a five-year-old child and student in Nice, France, with both ASD and anxiety. We have briefly described what ASD and anxiety are; we have also given a short empirical overview of ABA, EBP, and IU and have seen how, in combination, they are complementary conceptual frameworks for the management of anxiety in children with ASD. In addition, we have included some very basic—but effective—instructional accommodations, environmental accommodations, and assessment accommodations. As previously indicated, these strategies can be used both at home and at school to help Zoe generalize her behaviors in order to control her anxiety which, in her case, is linked to her ASD. However, we have not yet heard Zoe's own narrative telling us how she herself views successful family-school team communication. We will, therefore, conclude this case study by listening to her narrative.

A CONCLUDING WORD FROM ZOE

We have deliberately left Zoe's narrative until the end of this chapter. Why? It sometimes happens that parents and school staff alike become wrapped up in their own adult expectations, with a plethora of meeting dates and times, and get caught up in the details of who is implementing which strategy, or not. Yet, all the adults involved with Zoe need to remember that they are dealing with a vulnerable child who sees the world in her very own unique way. Therefore, we should never forget how the family-school team's joint work impacts her everyday life, whether positively or negatively. With this in mind, we will now present Zoe's view of her new world when the family-school team is working well together:

New friends . . . I want new friends . . . Mom told me that I will be making new friends. I'm going to the school for big kids. I'm a big girl now. I will whisper when I need to repeat a sentence from a cartoon over and over so that the other kids don't look at me like they sometimes do. Mom taught me to do this. I will try to control myself. I want new friends. I have to work and be nice. Mom said that if I am nice, I'll be able to stay in the big girls' school. I have to make sure not to talk to myself too loudly in the classroom. I must not bother Maîtresse or I'll be kicked out of my class, and I'll have to go to another school again. They say I am different, so I have to behave or I won't be allowed to stay with everyone. Who is this new woman next to me? She smells like perfume and her third finger has chipped nail polish. Will she fix it? Her nail polish is chipped. It's broken. She should fix it. She is nice, she talked to me, but I couldn't listen. I was looking at her chipped nail polish. Since I arrived, she has been very nice and the Directrice as well. I heard her say that she talked to my mom. Ooooh great! I see my notebook with Princess Ariel on it. I love this book. It is the same one as in the school for young kids. Now I know what she was asking me to do while I was looking at her nail. I will work like a big girl. I love being a big girl. Mom says that if I work well, I will have her phone when I come back home. I love playing on the phone. I love my new school. Everyone is nice and it seems they already know how to help me. I will be a big girl this year and I will get Maman's phone every day.

As can be seen, Zoe's narrative describes in simple yet powerful terms an example of what a successful strategy implementation by a family-school team may look like from the perspective of a five-year-old child with ASD and anxiety. On the other hand, it does not describe Zoe's hand and nail-biting, screaming, and other behaviors mentioned earlier in this case study which occur when strategies and communication are not quite so successful. Therefore, from our point of view, the advantages of a family-school team working together should be obvious to all for Zoe's sake, despite any reservations that parents, such as Mme C., or the school principal, such as Mme L., may initially have. It is our hope that you share this perspective as well after reading Zoe's view of her world.

BRIEF CRITICAL QUESTIONS

- Reflect on how to plan transitions from one activity to the next.
- Look for examples of "visual schedules for autism" on Google and design your own for a classroom activity. Reflect on tools that you could have in your classroom to help structure time and the environment.

REFLEXIVE RESPONSES

1. How would you introduce Zoe to the students in your classroom? How would you explain her needs and interests in order to facilitate her inclusion in the class?
2. Within your own classroom, how could you reorganize the seating arrangement to minimize distractions for children who have learning difficulties?
3. Based on space management strategies and content adaptation, what could you do to help an easily distracted child with ASD and anxiety complete a full sheet of exercises consisting of five different mathematical problems on the same page?
4. Alain is a child with ASD and anxiety. He has no intellectual challenges. However, he has been complaining that he is "useless and not good enough." What strategies could you use to help this child develop better self-esteem? Think about putting him in a position of success and about positive reinforcements.
5. Sophie is an eight-year-old girl with ADHD and anxiety who can focus on a task for only four minutes at a time. She is presented with a complex task that includes multiple steps that should take around ten minutes to complete. What strategies would you use to prevent the development of problem behaviors so as to help her succeed in completing what is asked of her?

REFERENCES

Abdelnour, H. (2019). *Teaching social skills to children on the autism spectrum through a peer-mediated intervention: A systematic literature review.* Unpublished Master's Thesis. Queen's University, Belfast.

American Psychiatric Association. (2013). *Diagnostic and statistical manual of mental disorders* (5th ed.). American Psychiatric Association. https://doi.org/10.1176/appi.books.9780890425596.

Bailey, J. S., & Burch, M. R. (2016). *Ethics for behavior analysts* (3rd ed.). Routledge-Taylor & Francis Group.

Boulter, C., Freeston, M., South, M., & Rodgers, J. (2014). Intolerance of uncertainty as a framework for understanding anxiety in children and adolescents with autism spectrum disorders. *Journal of Autism and Developmental Disorders, 44*(6), 1391–1402. https://doi.org/10.1007/s10803-013-2001-x.

Buhr, K., & Dugas, M. J. (2009). The role of fear of anxiety and intolerance of uncertainty in worry: An experimental manipulation. *Behaviour Research and Therapy, 47*(3), 215–223. https://doi.org/10.1016/j.brat.2008.12.004.

Cihak, D., Fahrenkrog, C., Ayres, K. M., & Smith, C. (2010). The use of video modeling via video iPod and a system of least prompts to improve transitional behaviors for students with autism spectrum disorders in the general education classroom. *Journal of Positive Behavior Interventions, 12*(3). https://doi.org/10.1177/1098300709332346.

Cohen, D. J., & Volkmar, F. R. (1997). *Handbook of autism and pervasive developmental disorders* (2nd ed.). Wiley.

Cooper, J. O., Heron, T. E., & Heward, W. L. (2014). *Applied behavior analysis* (2nd ed.). Pearson Education Limited.

Gingras, F. P., & Côté, C. (2016). La théorie et le sens de la recherche. In B. Gauthier & I. Bourgeois (Eds), *Recherche sociale. De la problématique à la collecte de données* (6th ed., pp. 103–128). Presses de l'Université du Québec.

Heflin, L. J., & Simpson, R. L. (1998). Interventions for children and youth with autism: Prudent choices in a world of exaggerated claims and empty promises. Part I: Intervention and treatment option review. *Focus on Autism and Other Developmental Disabilities, 13*(4), 194–211. https://doi.org/10.1177/108835769801300401.

Hillman, K., Dix, K., Kashfee, A., Lietz, P., Trevitt, J., O'Grady, E., Uljarević, M., Vivanti, G., & Hedley, D. (2020). Interventions for anxiety in mainstream school-aged children with autism spectrum disorder: A systematic review. *Campbell Systemic Reviews.* Advance online publication. https://doi.org/10.1002/cl2.1086.

Knight, V., Spriggs, A., & Sartini, E. (2014). Evaluating visual activity schedules as evidence-based practice for individuals with autism spectrum disorder. *Journal of Autism and Developmental Disorders, 45*, 157–178. https://doi.org/10.1007/s10803-014-2201-z.

Kulage, K. M., Goldberg, J., Usseglio, J., Romero, D., Bain, J. M., & Smaldone, A. M. (2020). How has DSM-5 affected autism diagnosis? A 5-year follow-up systematic literature review and meta-analysis. *Journal of Autism and Developmental Disorders, 50*, 2102–2127. https://doi.org/10.1007/s10803-019-03967-5.

Lin, A., Rangel, A., & Adolphs, R. (2012). Impaired learning of social compared to monetary rewards in autism. *Frontiers in Neuroscience, 6*, 143. https://doi.org/10.3389/fnins.2012.00143.

Lynch, C. (2019, June 3). Relaxation training for kids on the autism spectrum: 5 Essential modifications. *Psychology Today*. https://www.psychologytoday.com/ us/blog/autism-and-anxiety/201906/relaxation-training-kids-the-autism-spectrum.

O'Nions, E., Christie, P., Gould, J., Viding, E., & Happe, F. (2014). Development of the Extreme Demand Avoidance Questionnaire (EDAQ): Preliminary observations on a trait measure for pathological demand avoidance. *Journal of Child Psychology & Psychiatry*, *55*(7), 758–768. https://doi.org/10.1111/jcpp.12149.

Pellicano, E., & Burr, D. (2012). When the world becomes 'too real': A Bayesian explanation of autistic perception. *Trends in Cognitive Sciences*, *16*(10), 50410. https://doi.org/10.1016/j.tics.2012.08.009.

Pilkington, K., Kirkwood, G., Rampes, H., Cummings, M., & Richardson, J. (2007). Acupuncture for anxiety and anxiety disorders—A systematic literature review. *Acupuncture in Medicine*, *25*(1–2). https://doi.org/10.1136/aim.25.1-2.1.

Schuetze, M., Rohr, C. S., Dewey, D., McCrimmon, A., & Bray, S. (2017). Reinforcement learning in autism spectrum disorder. *Frontier of Psychology*. https://www.frontiersin.org/articles/10.3389/fpsyg.2017.02035/full.

Skinner, B. F. (2014). *Science and human behaviour*. Pearson Education.

Slocum, T. A., Detrich, R., Wilczynski, S. M., Spencer, T. D., Lewis, T., & Wolfe, K. (2014). The evidence-based practice of applied behavior analysis. *Association of Behaviour Analysis International*, *37*, 41–56. https://doi.org/10.1007/s40614 -014-0005-2.

Stuart, L., Grahame, V., Honey, E., & Freeston, M. (2020). Intolerance of uncertainty and anxiety as explanatory frameworks for extreme demand avoidance in children and adolescents.*Child and Adolescent Mental Health*. Advance online publication. https://doi.org/10.1111/camh.12336.

Tsai, L. (2012). Sensitivity and specificity: DSM-IV versus DSM-5 criteria for autism spectrum disorder. *The American Journal of Psychiatry*, *169*(10), 1009–1011. https://doi.org/10.1176/appi.ajp.2012.12070922.

Wigham, S., Rodgers, J., South, M., McConachie, H., & Freeston, M. (2015). The interplay between sensory processing abnormalities, intolerance of uncertainty, anxiety and restricted and repetitive behaviours in autism spectrum disorder. *Journal of Autism and Developmental Disorders*, *45*, 943–952. https://doi.org/10 .1007/s10803-014-2248-x.

Chapter 4

Case Story #4—Assisting a Student with Bipolar Disorder in West Africa

Margaret Janse van Rensburg and Olivia Atsin

THEORETICAL MODEL AND BACKGROUND

Making ethical decisions is at the heart of providing education that fosters positive mental health in students. Ethical decisions are often grounded in metaethics and standard prescriptions of right and wrong. In vivo, these ethical codes often prove unused or underused. The ethics of care identifies that people rely on one another and that ethical decisions are rooted in the caring responsibilities of attentiveness, responsibility, and competence. It is through dependency and vulnerability, inherent in the human condition, that moral and ethical persons develop. Lloyd (2010) outlines that there are four nonsequential phases within ethics of care: attentiveness through caring about, responsibility through taking care of, competence through caregiving, and responsiveness through care receiving. The ethics of care is pertinent in the following case study, about Winnie, a young girl from Côte d'Ivoire, who remains undiagnosed with bipolar disorder, because it outlines the need for her teacher to be attentive to her mood fluctuations, responsible through taking care of the situation in a classroom setting, competent in giving care to Winnie alone, and responsive through getting assistance from colleagues within the school.

WINNIE'S STORY

Winnie, a ten-year-old girl leaves for recess ecstatic and ready to play with her friends. She is the first one in line and is bouncing with enthusiasm waiting for the bell to ring. Fifteen minutes later, at the end of recess, Winnie comes back in, last in line, dragging her feet and head down. She slumps

41

down as she sits down. You realize that this has been happening a lot lately, Winnie being very energetic in one moment while at another moment she seems down and, well, depressed.

Along with this, she has been getting stomach aches almost daily and been asking to be sent home when she has been in this low-energy state. When she has good days and times, it seems that she is almost the most highly energetic student, but then there are those like today when she switches to sadness. Then, there are those days when she does not come at all, even more frequently this past month. You notice that on some days her face lightens up and she can be the most energetic student in class, while on others, she tends to be extremely moody and isolates.

You check in with Winnie, asking her if something happened at recess. She replies that she does not know what is wrong but she just feels really sad all of a sudden, that her tummy feels funny and that she wants to go home. In your school, the first step is to send a sick child to the infirmary. She does not seem in distress so you are hesitant to call her parents. Lately, she has not been performing well at school either, and her parents shared that they might suspect she is being "lazy" and "gets too easily distracted." You feel like the best choice or decision in this situation is to dismiss Winnie to go to the infirmary, and if she is sick, they can either help her with the illness or call her parents to pick her up.

Later that day, you check in with the school nurse about Winnie. The nurse tells you that this was similar to the other times Winnie has asked to be sent home. "I asked her what was wrong, she said she doesn't know. All she knows is that she doesn't feel good or happy. She complains of stomach aches sometimes, not always, but she is not physically ill. Sometimes the more I inquire she either stops herself from telling me the whole story or she just starts weeping. I think something more is going on." In consulting the nurse, you decide that the next step might be to contact a school psychologist to see if there are mental health reasons that Winnie may be facing these hardships.

In the society you live in, you are cognizant of the fact that mental illness is not really talked about openly, especially because many parents do not believe in mental illnesses or do not know how to handle children when they have mental health experiences or suffer trauma. The parents often believe that children are unaware of a lot of things. In addition, facilities for treatment or trained psychologists are a fairly scarce commodity while the encouraged or go-to method is community care and assistance.

A month later you are given information from the school psychologist that Winnie has been diagnosed with bipolar disorder. Bipolar disorder is a chronic affective disorder with recurrent episodes of mood fluctuations (Kleinman et al., 2003). Persons living with bipolar disorder can have impaired occupational functioning, a reduction health-related quality of life,

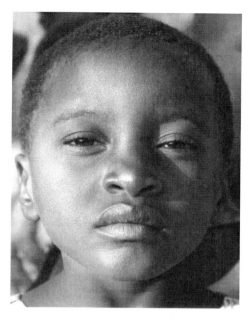

Figure 4.1   Winnie and living with bipolar disorder. Case Story #4. *Pixabay License.* https://pixabay.com/photos/child-face-african-africa-poverty-4617142/.

and are at a higher risk of suicide. While Kleinman et al. (2003) propose that bipolar disorder has a lifetime prevalence of approximately 1.3 percent, other literature speculates that persons living with bipolar make up 5–8 percent of the general population (Kessler et al., 2007; Severus & Bauer, 2013). Persons living with bipolar disorder may require inpatient treatment, outpatient treatment, other psychiatric and psychological services, as well as access to medical care (Geddes & Miklowitz, 2013; Kleinman et al., 2003). Persons living with bipolar disorder disproportionately experience stigmatization, which can have critical repercussions for their functioning, social support, and courses of illness. As a teacher who works with a student who lives with bipolar disorder, it is integral to use this information in creating educational and social experiences for the student to thrive.

BRIEF CRITICAL RESPONSE QUESTIONS

1. Winnie's parents are resistant to her seeing the school psychologist. Based on the Ethics of Care, what steps can you take to normalize the experience of seeing the school psychologist to Winnie's parents.

2. You hear a child saying that Winnie is a *psycho*. What can you say in this situation to destigmatize bipolar disorder while keeping Winnie's diagnosis confidential? How would you deal with this situation if it was a coworker speaking about Winnie in this way?
3. How would you approach interacting with Winnie in the future when she is displaying a low-energy state without pathologizing her, while being sensitive to her mental illness?

REFLECTIVE RESPONSE QUESTIONS

1. Have you ever called something or someone "bipolar"? How do you think using this term this way impacts stigmatization of the mental illness?
2. Families from different cultures may have different thoughts and feelings about mental health. How can you respect different cultural interpretations of mental health while keeping the needs of the child as a primary goal?
3. Are you open to integrating community care or assistance to your work? How would you approach integrating community care into your teaching?

STRATEGIES OF SUPPORT TO CONSIDER

- Work in collaboration with the school psychologist and nurse to decrease the amount of time that Winnie is spending in the infirmary during class hours. Be willing to offer accommodations for alternative methods of teaching and testing based on fluctuations in mood.
- When Winnie does spend time in the infirmary, it's important for her to understand that she does not have to feel ashamed or afraid. Let her know before she leaves that she can come back to class any time if she feels like it, even during recess.
- Provide time to listen to Winnie and allow her to express herself and listen to her too during the times when she feels sad or depressed without always jumping to give advices.
- Find creative ways for Winnie to express herself or just distract herself such as coloring books.
- Learn about the importance of community. Self-reflect on the following questions:
  - What does community mean to me?
  - Who is my community?

- ○ What things are required for community?
- ○ What could be the impact of a loving and supportive community?
- ○ Why is a loving and supportive community important?
- Promote a community within your classroom and school environment which is inclusive, nonjudgmental, and caring of all. Make respect and consent a cornerstone of the activities that you provide for your class.
- Speak to Winnie's parents about the importance of community. Assist the school psychologist in explaining the impacts of her mental illness on her learning and social relationships. Come up with strategies for Winnie's parents to learn more about the reality of mental illness, about bipolar disorder, learn how to support their child (in addition to community support if that's the route they want to take) now that they have this diagnosis.
- Take a nonjudgmental approach in speaking about mental health to the class. Allow for conversations surrounding mental health to normalize the experiences of all students. Be creative around how to approach the topic in class so children can really understand.
- Listen for any stigmatizing language used in the classroom setting. For example, if a student says, "This weather is so bipolar," be curious to the reasons they say that, and then explain that it is not appropriate to use that term in that way.
- Bring in survivors of mental illness into the class to speak about their experiences and/or show movies about successful persons with mental illness. This may increase a person's feelings of competency and ability to succeed, even with a diagnosis of bipolar disorder.
- Take a course in suicide intervention.

CONCLUSION

Children living with bipolar disorder have the capacity to learn and thrive in supportive educational settings. Approaching teaching using ethics of care in decision-making assists educators in being responsive to the needs of their students, while being open and willing to refer to others when they cannot provide adequate care. In the context of Côte d'Ivoire, mental health may be a suppressed topic in the classroom. Teachers have a responsibility to be attentive that their students may experience mental illness, to adapt their teaching for these students, and to promote acceptance of these students within their classroom, their schools, and in the child's family. Community support is integral in ensuring well-being for persons living with bipolar disorder. Other methods such as medication and therapeutic approaches may complement community, but are not always accessible or the best option for every child, especially in community-oriented environments. It is important to understand that there is no one-size-fits-all approach to mental illnesses. Providing avenues for a student to have a community in which people can hold space for the parents and the student to express themselves without any shame or judgment. Communities including people that the student can confide in, develop relationships with, and ultimately can trust. Overall, they offer options for a student in distress to reach out and be listening to in an active manner. Being alone can have detrimental consequences, and therefore an educator's role is to provide avenues for a student to create and feel supported by a community. When children reach a certain age, it is important to make them an integral part in the process of managing their mental illness so it could be easier to cope in the future, without feeling lost, helpless, or out of control.

LINKS TO RELEVANT ONLINE MATERIALS/VIDEOS

- LivingWorks—SafeTALK and ASIST provide simple tools for all people to bring up and prevent suicide: https://www.livingworks.net/
- International Bipolar Foundation: https://ibpf.org/
- International Society for Bipolar Disorders: https://www.isbd.org/
- Mental Health Commission of Canada. (2012). Together Against Stigma: Challenging How we see Mental Illness: https://www.mentalhealthcom mission.ca/sites/default/files/Stigma_Opening_Minds_Together_Against _Stigma_ENG_0.pdf
- Canadian Mental Health Association. (2001). Talking About Mental Illness: Teacher's Resource: https://www.camh.ca/-/media/files/guides-and -publications/tami-teachers-guide.pdf
- Child and Adolescent Bipolar Association (2007). Educating a Child with Bipolar Disorder: https://www.dbsalliance.org/pdfs/BMPN/edbrochure.pdf

REFERENCES

Geddes, J. R., & Miklowitz, D. J. (2013). Treatment of bipolar disorder. *Lancet, 381*(9879), 1672–1682. https://www.ncbi.nlm.nih.gov/pmc/articles/PMC3876031/.
Kessler, R. C., Akiskal, H. S., Ames, M., Birnbaum, H., Greenberg, P. E., Hirschfeld, R. M., & Wang, P. S. (2007). Considering the costs of bipolar depression. *Psychiatry & Behavioural Health Learning Network.* https://www.psychcongress .com/article/considering-costs-bipolar-depression.
Kleinman, L., Lowin, A., Flood, A., Gandhi, G., Edgell, E., & Reviki, D. (2003). Costs of bipolar disorder. *Pharmacoeconomics, 21*(9), 601–622. https://doi.org/10 .2165/00019053-200321090-00001.
Severus, E., & Bauer, M. (2013). Diagnosing bipolar disorders in DSM-5. *International Journal of Bipolar Disorders, 1,* 14. https://www.researchgate.net/publication /270653434_Diagnosing_bipolar_disorders_in_DSM-5.

Chapter 5

Case Story #5—"Being My Neighbor's Keeper"

Mental Health Challenges in Ghana

Magnus Mfoafo-M'Carthy and Jennie Beck

THEORETICAL MODEL AND BACKGROUND

Abeiku is a twelve-year-old junior high school student in a private institution located in Accra, Ghana. He is the eldest of four siblings. Teachers in his school, particularly his class teacher, Ms. B, have observed Abeiku exhibiting unusual behaviors over the past year. For example, the teachers have noticed that he is easily angered, he is very argumentative, and he rarely focuses on class activities. The teachers have shared these concerns with the school principal, Mr. C, who has met with Abeiku's mother, Mama Akua, on three occasions regarding his behavior. Though the mother, Mama Akua, acknowledges seeing changes in her son's behavior, she appears to be at a loss regarding how to access treatment or support for her son. Unfortunately, the school lacks the resources and the personnel to provide any support for Abeiku or the mother. Mama Akua mentioned to the principal, Mr. C., that she had discussed her son's condition with her pastor who has prayed for Abeiku and the family against any "demonic" or outside influences. Though the pastor continues to pray for the family, not much has changed from the perspectives of the mother and school authorities.

Mama Akua has been advised to either make an appointment for Abeiku to see a psychologist or a psychiatrist for support, but she worries about her inability to afford payment for the services. She also fears the community's perception of her son's condition and is wary of the attitudes toward Abeiku as he begins seeking treatment from a mental health specialist. The other worry is the limited number of mental health professionals in the country which makes it almost impossible to schedule an appointment with a specialist. The school authorities are not very familiar with the mental health system but decided to hire a psychologist on a part-time basis to provide support for Abeiku and other students going through similar challenges.

ABEIKU'S STORY

I arrived at school a bit early today and decided to spend a bit of time chatting with my mates sitting under the mango tree. As soon as I got there, I overheard John calling me names and making fun of me. As soon as he started calling me names, I got angry and felt the urge to punch him. I tackled and punched him a couple of times. The more I punched him, the more I felt the compulsion to keep hitting him. We were eventually separated, and I was called to the principal's office. Mr. C, the principal, accused me of being in the wrong, but I know I defended myself. What the principal said made me angry because he does not understand and did not want to hear my side of the story. I am angry, and I feel the world is not fair. I am not ready to talk to my teacher, even though he has asked me to join my colleagues in class. They keep threatening me with expulsion from the school. I am sick and tired of life and all that is going on. I might as well end it all and then you will be happy.

BRIEF RESPONSE

Despite the lack of knowledge about mental illness and the unwillingness to explore the topic by many Ghanaians and Africans as a whole, due to the stigma associated with it, it is necessary for the principal to have a conversation with Abeiku and address the issue of suicide. The teachers should find a way to provide support and guidance for Abeiku and his mother. Though the mother has tried to reach out to her pastor, she remains concerned about society's perception of the son's condition. There may be an opportunity for the school's psychologist to share concerns about mental health and the stigma associated with it to the school authorities.

The school could address these concerns about mental illness by empowering the psychologist to hold educational sessions with the students. In turn, this would address some of the challenges associated with mental health stigma in society. Issues to be addressed and discussed with the students could include their perception of mental illness and how that could be challenged by findings in contemporary research and discoveries in terms of medications that have shown to improve people's well-being. Thus, instead of seeing Abeiku as a danger and making fun of him by calling him names,

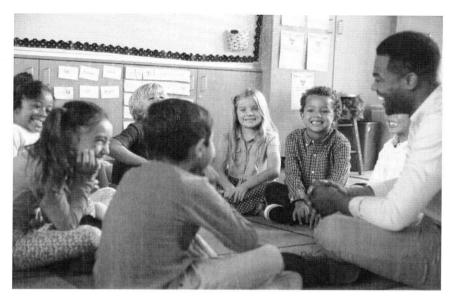

Figure 5.1 Facilitating educational sessions with students to support their friend, Abeiku. Case Story #5. *iStock—Standard License.* https://stock.adobe.com/images/elementary-school-kids-and-teacher-sit-cross-legged-on-floor/104937752?prev_url=detail.

they may learn to be supportive of him. How can the students be taught empathy regarding mental health?

REFLECTIVE RESPONSE QUESTIONS

1. You have been informed by the principal that Abeiku has threatened to attempt suicide. However, he has been asked by the principal to come to class. How would you react? What steps would you take to accommodate Abeiku?
2. Could you name, describe, and explain supports you would put in place to support Abeiku? Why do you think these supports are necessary?
3. How would you explain to other students in the class what is going on with Abeiku? What steps would you take to make Abeiku feel safe? What steps would you take to foster a safe environment for all students in the class?

MENTAL HEALTH STIGMA IN GHANA

There is a 98 percent treatment gap of Ghanaians who have severe or moderate to mild mental illnesses. This means that only 60,000 of the estimated

2.82 million persons in Ghana who have mental illness are receiving psychiatric treatment (WHO, 2007). Ghana's government health budget is quite low at 1.4 percent, which amounts to $31 per person per year, and a minuscule 0.5 percent of this funding goes toward mental health. Though the World Bank classifies Ghana as a low-income country, the amount of government expenditure on mental health treatment and resources is not justifiable (Jacob et al., 2007). Barke et al. (2011), however, argues that the stigmatization of mental illness in Ghana is why so few resources are given to mental health research and psychiatric hospitals. A study conducted in 1975 analyzed perceptions of mental illness by Ghanaian high school and college students. Results indicated that 57.9 percent of respondents believed mental illness brings shame on one's family, while 57.3 percent of respondents believed it was best to keep one's mental illness a secret. Even a larger majority at 78.9 percent of participants believed that patients with mental illness in hospitals are like children, and 71.8 percent believed that anyone hospitalized from a mental illness should not have the right to vote (Ngissah, 1975).

Since Ngissah's study conducted in 1975, there has been a slight improvement in the overall perceptions of mental illness by Ghanaian citizens; however, the detrimental effects of stigma against the mentally ill remain pervasive. Barke et al. (2011) explain that the level of stigma found in Ngissah's (1975) study is very comparable to sentiments expressed today. A study by Franke et al. examined the attitudes and desire of young Ghanaians to remain socially distant from people with symptoms of schizophrenia and depression (Franke et al., 2019). A respondent's decision to be socially distant from a person who has a mental illness included: not offering them a room to rent, not accepting them as a colleague or neighbor, not allowing them to take care of their children, and so on. Results indicated that the more severe the mental illness is and the closer the participant and their family are to this individual, the more likely a participant would want to remain distant from the person with mental illness. For example, 51.6 percent of respondents would accept someone with schizophrenia as a neighbor and 63.3 percent would accept someone with depression as a neighbor; however, only 23 percent of participants would marry into the family of someone who has schizophrenia and 30.4 percent would marry into the family of someone who has depression (Franke et al., 2019).

Many members of the Ghanaian public believe that mental illnesses are caused by supernatural and spiritual influences (Mfoafo-M'Carthy & Soussou, 2017). These views are often held by policy makers and sometimes held by health professionals, making very difficult the implementation of anti-stigma campaigns and educational opportunities that explain the psychosocial and biological origins of mental illness (Omar et al., 2010). Due to the lack of government-implemented mental health resources and the stigma associated with utilizing these psychiatric services, approximately 70–80 percent of Ghanaians use traditional medicine as a form of treatment (Barke et al., 2011). Quinn (2007) reports that due to many believing mental illness is related to supernatural powers, utilizing traditional healers as opposed to hospital treatments carries less stigma. Culturally, specific explanations of mental illness associated with higher rates of acceptance can be attributed to the lack of formal education on mental health and mental illness in Ghana's school curriculums.

In the School of Social Work at the University of Ghana, for instance, mental health theory is missing from the curriculum of the bachelor of social work program. Although students can take courses related to mental health at the master's level, most students do not even take these courses, and sometimes not even a single student is registered for those electives (Gilbert & Dako-Gyeke, 2018). Social workers are supposed to advocate for the marginalized; however, if a majority of Ghana's social workers are not interested in studying mental health, who fights for this excluded population? Perceptions of mental illness in Ghana can be changed through education, yet students should be taught about mental health and mental illness from a younger age to reduce stigma and misunderstanding.

HOW STIGMA AFFECTS THOSE WITH MENTAL ILLNESS AND THEIR FAMILIES

Barke et al. (2011) conducted a study to explore the perceived stigma of Ghanaians with mental illness. Using surveys completed by patients in psychiatric hospitals across the nation, the findings indicate most of the participants feeling devalued and excluded socially. Furthermore, most of the participants anticipated difficulty in finding work upon discharge from the hospital. These findings are in line with other studies (Franke et al., 2019; Mfoafo-M'Carthy & Grischow, 2020), signifying the exclusionary measures of the mentally ill that are embedded in Ghanaian culture are felt by those who are ill and have a deep impact on their well-being. This can result in self-stigmatization, which can potentially have a huge negative influence on an individual's health outcomes. Self-stigmatization is related to low self-esteem and can trigger more severe psychiatric symptoms, potentially leading to an increased risk of suicide (Gyamfi et al., 2018).

Age plays a large role in self-stigmatization. According to Tally (2009), although it is common for adolescents to be confused or angry in response to having a mental illness, they tend to report less self-stigmatization. Individuals who believed the discrimination they were facing is illegitimate and who rejected the exclusion they experienced were more resilient to stigma. In the case of Ghana and other countries where stigma of mental illness is pervasive, having the strength to reject the attitudes of most members of one's community is nearly impossible. Gyamfi et al.'s (2018) study examining self-stigma of outpatients in a psychiatric hospital found that most participants shared and accepted the perspective of their illness held by their communities. Many felt that their poor mental health was their own fault, citing punishment for sin or supernatural powers. This often resulted in self-isolation through fear of anticipated discrimination, including choosing not to pursue their education or apply for a job (Gyamfi et al., 2018).

Due to insufficient mental health resources in Ghana, many family members take on the responsibility of looking after their loved ones who are sick. Not only does the burden of caregiving affect the well-being of the family members, but the stigma these families must endure makes it even more challenging (Ae-Ngibise et al., 2015; Mfoafo-M'Carthy & Grischow, 2020). Ae-Ngibise et al. (2015) conducted a study to explore through qualitative interviewing the experiences of caregivers of people living with serious mental illnesses. Many participants reported feelings of emotional distress, particularly involving the embarrassment they faced due to the stigma and fear others have of their loved one.

Tawiah et al.'s (2015) study, which reports on the stigma faced by patients in a psychiatric hospital and their caregivers, provided interesting results in terms of caregivers' perspectives of mental illness. Findings indicate that most of the patients and their caregivers believed the causes of mental illness are predominately biological. These families make a strong effort to reject the stigma they face in their communities and have developed social strategies to cope with the exclusion (Tawiah et al., 2015). These results provide a more optimistic lens of the effects of stigma in the country compared to the various other studies analyzed (Barke et al., 2011; Gyamfi et al., 2018; Quinn, 2007). Most of the patients and their caregivers in psychiatric hospitals who participated in this study preferred biomedical treatment as opposed to the traditional practices that are common in Ghana (Tawiah et al., 2015). Although one may assume this rejection of stigma and commitment to scientific treatment of mental illness is associated with higher levels of education, only 11 percent of participants had postsecondary education (Tawiah et al., 2015). Most participants in Ae-Nigibise et al.'s (2015) study exhibited similar perspectives of stigma in Ghanaian culture. Caregivers in the study indicated that education and awareness of what mental illness is, how it is caused, and how it can be treated are essential to stop the taunting and exclusion of the mentally ill.

Both Ae-Nigibise et al.'s (2015) and Tawiah et al.'s (2015) studies explore the experiences of family members who are committed to supporting their loved ones despite the immense burden of caregiving and facing stigma in their community. This, however, is easier said than done. Many who choose to seek treatment in psychiatric hospitals for their mental illness end up being abandoned by their families once they are discharged. This trend is so common that a special ward in a psychiatric hospital has been created for patients who have been rejected from their families due to stigma (Barke et al., 2011). The decision of families to abandon their loved ones due to stigma can be compared to Gyamfi et al.'s (2018) study on self-stigmatization. It is so difficult to ignore the beliefs of one's community and listen to the science when stigma is so common, pervasive, and entrenched over generations. This can explain the immense congestion of those who have been abandoned in psychiatric hospitals (Tawiah et al., 2015). It is understandably difficult to sacrifice one's inclusion in the community to take on the burden of caregiving in an unsupportive environment.

HOW STIGMA AFFECTS MENTAL HEALTH SERVICES IN GHANA

As stigma of mental health is so pervasive in Ghana, it has an ability to seep into government health policies, ultimately determining the effectiveness of mental health resources and the quality of care given by professionals (Sottie et al., 2018). Omar et al. (2010) explain that mental health policies in Ghana are "weak, in draft form or are non-existent; furthermore, they are poorly implemented" (p. 7). Since many policy makers and even health professionals believe that mental illness is caused by supernatural power, the development of policies and assignment of resources is given very low priority (Omar et al., 2010). The author explains that it is not only the lack of attention to policies themselves, but there is also an absence of structure and programs to ensure successful implementation of the policies. Policy actors who are experts in the field of mental health are also rarely consulted in Ghana. This results in a one-sided and narrow perspective which often blames the mentally ill for their condition, thus signifying the low priority of resources (Omar et al., 2010).

This lack of resources devoted to mental health affects the quality of the education and training of the professionals in this field, ultimately affecting the level of care received by the patients. For example, a report on Ghana's mental health system created by the government concluded that social workers in the area of mental health did not have specific mental health training prior to working with this population (Roberts, 2013). The report indicates that in 2011, only twenty-one social workers were working in mental health services in Ghana and out of those twenty-one, none had more than one year of training in working with individuals with mental illness (Roberts, 2013).

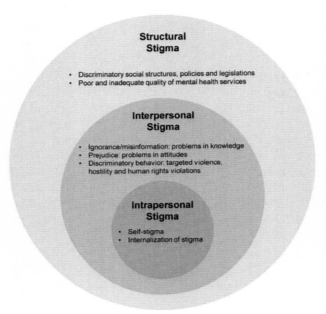

Figure 5.2   Types of stigma. Adapted from Afzal et al. (2021). Case Story #5. *Reducing the stigma of mental health disorders with a focus on low- and middle-income countries.* Asian Journal of Psychiatry, *58.* https://doi.org/10.1016/j.ajp.2021.102601. https://www.sciencedirect.com/science/article/pii/S1876201821000575.

Even Ghanaians studying mental health in postsecondary education are tentative to use mental health resources. Andoh-Arthur et al. (2015) analyzed the help-seeking intentions among university students in Ghana through cross-sectional surveys. Interestingly, it was discovered that students studying psychology were unlikely to seek counseling despite the assumption that this population would have learned about the value and importance of seeking psychological help if needed. This demonstrates a disconnect between implementing theory into practice (Andoh-Arthur et al., 2015). The study signifies the potential mistrust and disbelief in psychiatric treatment held by many professionals in Ghana working with mentally ill patients.

Adjorlolo et al. (2018) conveyed similar findings through an exploration of the attitudes of mental health professionals working with mentally ill offenders in Ghana. Results of the study indicated that the opinions of the mental health nurses regarding mental illness significantly predicted their treatment toward the offenders. Those who punished the offenders more frequently tended to have negative attitudes toward mental illness. Those who had practiced nursing for over six years also demonstrated a lack of sympathy and an increase in anger toward the offenders (Adjorlolo et al., 2018).

Interestingly, an unpublished study previously conducted by the contributor found that 46 percent of mental health professionals participating in the study believed that mental illness is caused by supernatural forces. This contributes to the argument that despite the profession, background, or education of an individual, and despite being educated and trained to look to science for answers, the power of stigma can sway one's opinions of mental illness (Adjorlolo et al., 2018).

WHAT IS BEING DONE TO FIGHT THE STIGMA

Educational and awareness campaigns of the biological and psychosocial origins of mental illness are necessary in Ghana. Despite the various studies of the issues stigma causes in the country, it is important to also explore the recent improvements of the mental health system and the organizations that are committed to fighting the stigma. In response to the many patients who have been abandoned by their families for seeking psychiatric treatment, a repatriation initiative was organized in 2011 to reunite patients with other family members and friends so they could be discharged and return home. Sending patients back home has the potential to greatly reduce the stigma by normalizing their presence and participation in society (Fournier, 2011). Before 2000, there were no nongovernmental organizations (NGO) in Ghana that focused on mental health; however, with awareness stemming from many mental health workers, organizations that aim to fight the stigma and educate the population have been on the frontlines of changing Ghana's perspective on mental illness (Fournier, 2011).

Mental Health Society of Ghana (MEHSOG) is a grassroots association aimed at supporting Ghanaians with mental illness and their caregivers while spreading awareness of mental health to stop the stigma. The organization has engaged the media to educate the public to use appropriate words and language when describing those with mental illness. Their efforts are manifested through seminars and workshops which focus on cultivating respect for people with mental health issues (MEHSOG, 2017).

Basic Needs Ghana is an organization which works to empower Ghanaians with mental illness and their families by targeting public opinion and government health policies related to mental health care in the nation. One of the projects the organization is running is a one-year initiative which aims to improve the mental health education of young adults and spread awareness of available mental health resources. This program is led by school mental health clubs which collaborate with teachers to develop student-led activities, information sessions, and awareness events (Basic Needs, 2020).

There are other NGOs based in Ghana which fight against the mental health stigma and support those with mental illness in the country; however, there are very few grassroots organizations where collective action is organized at the local level. While Basic Needs is a wonderful international NGO and their chapter in Ghana does great work, their model of care was developed by the chapter in the United Kingdom (Basic Needs, 2020). Considering that the mental health system and stigma surrounding mental illness are vastly different in the United Kingdom compared to Ghana, applying the same approach to collective action might not be as effective. For a better understanding and insights into mental health, organizations must engage in educating the populace to have a better understanding of the stigma associated with the illness and its impact on our society. This educational approach could be adopted by taking into consideration the unique culture, practices, and needs of the people.

STRATEGIES TO SUPPORT

It would be important for the school to make the effort to provide support for Abeiku. This could be in the form of a resource teacher or a special education instructor who would be able to guide him in the classroom and his interactions. In addition, Abeiku and his family could benefit from the support of a counselor. Though such services are rare in Ghanaian schools, it would be recommended that schools make such services available to students. As we already know, early intervention regarding mental health issues among children goes a long way to alleviate future challenges and costs families may incur. Abeiku's family could also benefit from the support of their extended family, pastor, and professional counseling.

CONCLUSION

Mental health challenges among school children is a global phenomenon that requires attention. In the global South, much attention is not given to mental health issues which tend to worsen as children grow older without medical or psychosocial intervention. It is noted that the reason why policy makers and government agencies do not pay much attention or take steps to mitigate these challenges are due to stigma and discriminatory attitudes associated with mental health issues. It is imperative that government leaders develop the political will to initiate measures that would ensure children are provided with adequate health care to enable them cope with psychological challenges/ trauma they may incur. Though there are several nongovernmental agencies

(NGOs) providing mental health services, it is realized that finding ways to address stigma and discriminatory practices in Ghana would make a huge difference.

LINKS TO RELEVANT ONLINE MATERIALS/VIDEOS

- Deconstructing Stigma: https://deconstructingstigma.org/home-of-brains -ghana
- United Nations Africa Renewal: https://www.un.org/africarenewal/news/ covid-19-halting-crucial-mental-health-services-africa-who-survey
- United Nations Association-Ghana (UNA-GH)—World Mental Health Day: https://www.unagh.org/world-mental-health-awareness-day/#

REFERENCES

Adjorlolo, S., Abdul-Nasiru, I., Chan, H. C., & Bambi, L. E. (2018). Mental health professionals' attitudes toward offenders with mental illness (insanity acquittees) in Ghana. *International Journal of Offender Therapy and Comparative Criminology*, *62*(3), 629–654. https://doi.org/10.1177/0306624X16666802.

Ae-Ngibise, K. A., Doku, V. C. K., Asante, K. P., & Owusu-Agyei, S. (2015). The experience of caregivers of people living with serious mental disorders: A study from rural Ghana. *Global Health Action*, *26957*. https://doi.org/10.3402/gha.v8 .26957.

Andoh-Arthur, J., Asante, K. O., & Osafo, J. (2015). Determinants of psychological help-seeking intentions of university students in Ghana. *International Journal of Advanced Counselling*, *37*, 330–345. https://doi.org/10.1007/s10447 -015-9247-2.

Barke, A., Nyarko, S., & Klecha, D. (2011). The stigma of mental illness in southern Ghana: Attitudes of the urban population and patients' views. *Social Psychiatry Psychiatric Epidemiology*, *46*, 1191–1202. https://doi.org/10.1007/s00127-010 -0290-3.

Basic Needs. (2020). *Basic needs – Ghana*. https://basicneedsghana.org/how-we -work/.

Fournier, O. A. (2011). The status of mental health care in Ghana, West Africa and signs of progress in the Greater Accra Region. *Berkeley Undergraduate Journal*, *24*(3), 8–32. https://doi.org/10.5070/B3243007890.

Franke, M. L., Lersner, U., Essel, O. Q., Adorjan, K., Schomerus, G., Gomez-Carrillo, A., TamTa, T. M., Boge, K., Mobashery, M., Dettling, M., Diefenbacher, A., Angermeyer, M. C., & Hahn, E. (2019). The relationship between causal beliefs and desire for social distance towards people with schizophrenia and depression: Results from a survey of young Ghanaian adults. *Psychiatry Research*, *271*, 220–225. https://doi.org/10.1016/j.psychres.2018.11.030.

Gilbert, D. J., & Dako-Gyeke, M. (2018). Lack of mental health career interest among Ghanaian social work students: Implications for social work education in Ghana. *Social Work Education, 37*(5), 665–676. https://doi.org/10.1080/02615479.2018.1447102.

Gyamfi, S., Hegadoren, K., & Park, T. (2018). Individual factors that influence experiences and perceptions of stigma and discrimination towards people with mental illness in Ghana. *International Journal of Mental Health Nursing, 27,* 368–377. https://doi.org/10.1111/inm.12331.

Jacob, K., Sharan, P., Mirza, I., Garrido-Cumbrera, M., Seedat, S., Mari, J., Sreenivas, V., & Saxena, S. (2007). Mental health systems in countries: Where are we now? *Lancet, 370,* 1061–1077. https://doi.org/10.1016/S0140-6736(07)61241-0.

Mental Health Society of Ghana. (2017, October 18). *Educating the public to increase interest in psychosocial disability issues to reduce stigma.* https://www.mehsog.org/2017/10/18/educating-the-public-to-increase-interest-in-psychosocial-disability-issues-to-reduce-stigma/.

Mfoafo-M'Carthy, M., & Grischow, J. (2020) "Being heard": The socio-economic impact of psychiatric care on patients and caregivers in Ghana. *International Social Work.* Advance online publication. https://doi.org/10.1177%2F0020872820962177.

Mfoafo-M'Carthy, M., & Sossou, M. (2017). Stigma, discrimination, and social exclusion of the mentally ill: The case of Ghana. *Journal of Human Rights and Social Work.* Advance online publication. https://doi.org/10.1007/s41134-017-0043-2.

Ngissah, P. (1975). *A comparative study of attitudes towards mental illness.* MA Thesis. California State University, California.

Omar, M. A., Green, A. T., Bird, P. K., Mirzoev, T., Flisher, A. J., Kigozi, F., Lund, C., Mwanza, J., & Ofori-Atta, A. L. (2010). Mental health policy process: A comparative study of Ghana, South Africa, Uganda and Zambia. *International Journal of Mental Health Systems, 4*(24), 1–10. https://doi.org/10.1186/1752-4458-4-24.

Quinn, N. (2007). Beliefs and community responses to mental illness in Ghana: The experiences of family carers. *International Journal of Social Psychiatry, 53,* 175–188. https://doi.org/10.1177/0020764006074527.

Roberts, M., Asare, J. B., Morgan, C., Adjase, E. T., & Osei, A. (2013). The mental health system in Ghana. *Ministry of Health: Republic of Ghana.* Advance online publication. https://doi.org/10.1177/0020764006074527.

Sottie, C., Mfoafo-M'Carthy, M., & Moasun, F. (2018). Graduate social work students' perceptions and attitude toward mental illness: Implications for practice in developing countries. *Social Work in Mental Health, 16*(5). https://doi.org/10.1080/15332985.2018.1448325.

Tally, M. (2009). Self-labeling and its effects among adolescents diagnosed with mental disorders. *Social Science & Medicine, 68,* 570–578. https://doi.org/10.1016/j.socscimed.2008.11.003.

Tawiah, P. E., Adongo, P. B., & Aikins, M. (2015). Mental health-related stigma and discrimination in Ghana: Experience of patients and their caregivers. *Ghana Medical Journal, 49*(1), 30–36. https://doi.org/10.4314/gmj.v49i1.6.

World Health Organization. (2007). *Ghana: A very progressive mental health law.* https://www.who.int/mental_health/policy/country/ghana/en/.

Chapter 6

Case Story #6—How Reading Gaps Impact a Young Child's Wellness in Canada

Jeffrey MacCormack

THEORETICAL MODEL AND BACKGROUND

For the following case study of Sophia, a Grade-4 student who has been having a difficult fall term, a model of self-efficacy has been utilized. This model recognizes that, while specific learning interventions are necessary for some students who have difficulty reading, the first challenge may be to persuade the student that they *can* improve. Students like Sophia may be experiencing a phenomenon called learned helplessness. As we know from Seligman and Maier's studies of canine responses, animals and humans do not do well when there is no way to stop bad things from happening. In their famous experiments, Seligman and Maier hurt dogs with electric shocks. For some dogs, the dog could press a lever to stop the shock and for other dogs, there was no way to stop the shock. With no way to avoid the shock, dogs would lay on the floor and whimper while they were being hurt; even when they had a way to stop the shocks, they were unwilling to try. In some ways, Sophia may be feeling like those dogs who cannot stop the shock. Sophia has some painful experiences trying to read and she is unwilling to continue to try. In short, Sophia has a self-efficacy problem: she doesn't believe she can improve. According to Bandura, there are four ways to help someone improve their self-efficacy. Verbal persuasion is usually what teachers try first ("Of course you can be successful! Keep trying"). Unfortunately, verbal persuasion is not very effective on its own. Sophia's self-efficacy is also influenced by her physiological states (depression and anxiety make it hard to maintain a sense of well-being). Another way to improve self-efficacy is watching others be successful, something Bandura called vicarious experiences. In this case, watching others read well may reinforce Sophia's belief that she is not capable. The fourth way to improve self-efficacy may be the best fit for Sophia: performance outcomes. After so many "shocking" failures, Sophia needs some wins under her belt. An effective teacher should be able to support Sophia by breaking the larger skills (reading with automaticity) into smaller constituent tasks, allowing Sophia to develop some fundamental skills and improving her sense of accomplishment and capacity.

SOPHIE'S STORY

Your colleague Mrs. Tremblay (Grade-4 teacher) came into your classroom to ask you for some advice about her student Sophia. She told you that one of her first clues that there was a problem with Sophia was the way she walked to school. At the beginning of the year, Sophia skipped alongside her older brother Jackson like the embodiment of enthusiasm, stopping only when an insect or a bird caught her eye. Other than her occasional stops to investigate butterflies or poke at squishy bugs, she seemed to be in a hurry to get to her Grade-3 classroom. By October, there was a noticeable change. After Thanksgiving break, Sophia's skip was gone, and by November, Sophia walked to school shuffling her feet in a way that suggested she never wanted to arrive.

Mrs. Tremblay became increasingly worried until, as she was cleaning up for winter break, she finally had some time to reflect on Sophia's situation. Mrs. Tremblay reviewed her anecdotal records from the first term and copied out the mentions of Sophia that seemed most relevant. As she passed you her notes, she said, "I know that reading has been a challenge, but we've been working on it."

09/15 . . . On day 3 of literacy centers, Sophia refused to read during independent reading center. She was getting emotional. I had started everyone off with a grade-2-level reader, so I was surprised she was having difficulty. I came over to help her and, with only a few prompts ("skip a word you don't know and come back to it," I told her), she started reading again. Or I assume she was reading. At least she was quiet. She is going to have to learn to work independently because grade 3 has a lot more independent work than the earlier grades do.

09/29 . . . Today was presentations of our novel studies. Sophia said her book was a graphic novel, but it was a comic book, no longer than 25 pages. Her presentation of the content was quite comprehensive, however. She shared some genuinely insightful points about the characters, but there was no way she got all of that from a comic book. She must have seen the movie.

10/04 . . . Small group reading today. Sophia became really emotional. She was crying when it came around to her turn. I asked her what the problem was. She said her stomach hurt.

10/26 . . . I finally got Sophia to read a sentence to me ("Mr. Lee spent three years carving his chair out of one piece of red oak"). Each word was a struggle. She read "chair" like this "see-ha, see-ha, no, no, cha, cha, cha, aye, aye, ire, cha-aye-ire, cha-aye-ire, chair." By the end of the reading, I asked her "why do you think Mr. Lee took so much time carving?" She looked at me, completely perplexed "Who is Mr. Lee?"

11/05 . . . Re: call to Sophia's parents. I couldn't get a hold of the family because the phone message said the mailbox was full. I wanted to tell the family that Sophia has been struggling a little in reading, especially during independent work, but her outburst in science today seemed to be a sign that her difficulties are spreading to other subjects. I told them that Sophia should not be saying "no, I'm just stupid" because those statements disrupt the class.

11/22 . . . The substitute teacher said that Sophia had a hard time during Reading Buddies time (teamed with the kindergarten class). "We can just look at the pictures and make up the story together," Sophia said to the kindergarten student. "I'm not a reader. That's just not my thing."

12/11 . . . This is the fourth day Sophia was absent in December, so I checked her attendance for the term. Sophia was present every day in September, absent four times in October, and absent eight times in November. At this rate, Sophia is going to miss almost twenty days over one term.

BRIEF CRITICAL RESPONSE QUESTIONS

1. Developing a habit of taking anecdotal notes of the day's events is an excellent strategy for teachers, but it can be hard to incorporate note taking into the busy teaching day. Browse online strategies for anecdotal note taking and find one that might work for you.
2. Like Sophia, who has already decided that she is "not a reader," students who experience difficulty reading with automaticity may feel helpless in their efforts to improve. How might you change Sophia's view of herself?
3. Reading programs in Grade 3 tend to emphasize comprehension skills over decoding skills, which often means that Grade-3 students who still have difficulty decoding are at a double disadvantage. What are the benefits and disadvantages of using high interest/easy reader texts, like comic books, for students like Sophia?

REFLECTIVE RESPONSE QUESTIONS

1. Communication between home and school is an important step in helping students like Sophia, but healthy two-way communication requires
   more of an effort than leaving a message on a phone machine. What
   should Mrs. Tremblay do next to facilitate and support home/school
   communication?
2. Use peer-reviewed literature and professional resources to identify and
   explain two strategies you could use to help Sophia learn to read.
3. Sophia would likely benefit from some one-on-one conversations with
   her teacher, but it may not be clear how to begin. How would you initiate
   those discussions? Explain your plan to get Sophia to open up.
4. There may be many reasons why Sophia's stomach hurts at school (e.g.,
   medical issues), but stomach pains are often symptoms of stress. How
   would you go about helping Sophia with her stomach pain?

STRATEGIES OF SUPPORT TO CONSIDER

- Connect with Sophia's parents. Reading programs at school will be more
  effective if they are transferred to the home as well.
- Keep a record of progress. Sophia can keep a journal of her reading level
  and books she read.
- Continue the conversation. Checking in with Sophia during student/teacher
  conferences can provide regular feedback, which will help Sophia feel like
  she is on a team.
- Learn more about resilience. Research people who succeeded in spite of
  failing at first (e.g., Larry Page cofounded Google in spite of early setbacks;
  Thierry Henry scored 228 goals for Arsenal, but didn't score any during his
  first 8 matches).

CONCLUSION

Considering Sophia's emotional state, supporting her will require a two-
pronged approach.

1. There is no doubt that one priority in supporting Sophia must be direct
   reading support. As Mrs. Tremblay suggested, reading has been a challenge for Sophia. While Sophia seems to be having more difficulty than

her peers at reading, reading difficulties are common for students in Grade 3. Comprehension is often a problem for students who are not able to read with automaticity because their cognitive resources are focused on decoding, instead of understanding the message. Sophia is going to need some deliberate and specific reading support from someone who understands the difficulties she faces. That said, Sophia is going to need more than direct support in reading.

2. The second priority in the two-prong approach to helping Sophia relates to her emotional well-being. It appears that Sophia has given up on herself in terms of being able to read. Instead of talking to her teacher about her reading difficulties, it appears that Sophia has been seeking work-around strategies for her reading tasks (watching movie and reading comic books, instead of reading novel study). Sophia's statement that she is "not a reader" is a red flag that she may be experiencing learned helplessness. When used to describe students, learned helplessness means that students feel powerless to make meaningful changes in their situation. As in Sophia's case, students with learned helplessness feel like they have done their best and were still unable to be successful.

While it may be tempting to think of Sophia's emotional well-being as less related to her academic work than her reading practice, the two approaches are deeply connected. Until Sophia *believes* that she can improve, she may not be willing to exert the effort she needs to be successful. Considering how often we tell students "practice makes progress" and "work hard to be successful," it should be no surprise that when students are unable to accomplish something their peers can do easily, those students are prone to feelings of shame. Students who feel shame tend to be less motivated to work hard (Weiner, 1985). Students in Sophia's situation may decide that, by not trying hard, they are protected from failure; after all, the reasoning goes, wouldn't it be easier to fail because of lack of effort than to fail because of lack of ability?

So, how can we help Sophia? According to Dweck (2015), the author of *Mindset: The New Psychology of Success*, helping Sophia requires that we help her adopt a growth mindset, the belief that intelligence can be developed. Sounds good, right? Well, the danger in *only talking* about growth mindset is that, when used along, verbal persuasion can worsen Sophia's situation. She has already tried (very hard!) to read, so reenforcing the message that her difficulties are her fault (lack of effort) would not be helpful. Remember that growth mindset requires more than applying more effort. Growth mindset

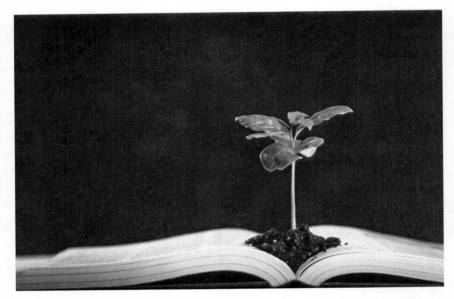

Figure 6.1. Growth mindset is only possible with new strategies and guided practice. Case Story #6. *iStock—Standard License.* https://stock.adobe.com/ca/images/本と植物/122314432?prev_url=detail.

requires new strategies and guided practice with feedback (Dweck, 2015). Additionally, anyone who wants to help Sophia first needs to gain her trust. In my experience, those conversations can be positive if the teacher emphasizes that learning to read is a partnership.

Sophia needs to know that

1. many people have difficulty reading in Grade 3,
2. many people who have difficulty reading in Grade 3 go on to read perfectly well later on,
3. there are heaps of reading strategies that they can work together, and
4. Sophia and the teacher are a team.

Supporting students like Sophia require a consideration of the students' sense of safety and well-being. Think back to the last time you tried to do something that was initially beyond your capacity and you'll agree that learning can be a scary thing. Trying hard at something makes us vulnerable to negative self-referential emotions like shame and guilt. For students like Sophia, she needs to be persuaded that there is nothing wrong if the process of learning something is effortful and time consuming.

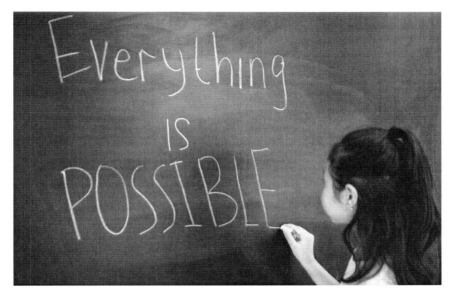

Figure 6.2. Trust between child and teacher supports risk-taking and growth. Case Story #6. *iStock—Standard License.* https://stock.adobe.com/ca/images/female-student -writing-text-of-everything-is-possible/282021585?prev_url=detail.

LINKS TO RELEVANT ONLINE MATERIALS/VIDEOS

- Seligman's Learned Helplessness: https://www.youtube.com/watch ?v=jEO3sJdoNV8
- Motivation as Self-Efficacy: https://socialsci.libretexts.org/Bookshelves/ Education_and_Professional_Development/Book%3A_Educational_Psy-chology_(Seifert_and_Sutton)/06%3A_Student_Motivation/6.06%3A_ Motivation_as_Self-Efficacy
- Early Reading Strategy: http://www.edu.gov.on.ca/eng/document/reports/ reading/effective.html

REFERENCES

Dweck, C. (2015). Carol Dweck revisits the growth mindset. *Education Week*, *35*(5), 20–24. https://www.edweek.org/leadership/opinion-carol-dweck-revisits -the-growth-mindset/2015/09.

Weiner, B. (1985). An attributional theory of achievement motivation and emotion. *Psychological Review*, *92*(4), 548–573. https://doi.org/10.1037/0033-295X.92.4.548.

Chapter 7

Case Story #7—PHOENIX

An Indigenous Learner

Gus Hill

LOCATION OF CONTRIBUTOR

Aaniin, Waase-Gaaboo Ndizhnikaaz, Anishnaabe Endaw, Obadjiwaan miinwaa Bawating Ndoonjibaa. Cambridge Endayaan. Hello, my spirit name is Waase-Gaaboo, and the name that I have been called for my whole life is Gus Hill. I am of Ojibwe, British and French ancestry, I grew up in Batchawana Bay, and Sault Ste. Marie, Ontario. My ancestors come from the North Shore of Lake Huron and the Eastern Shore of Lake Superior, in Ontario. I live with my family in Cambridge, Ontario. It is important for me to introduce myself in this way because it honors and respects my ancestors.

INTRODUCTION/BACKGROUND

I use the term "Indigenous" throughout this case study to denote First Nations, Metis, and Inuit/Innu people who are the original inhabitants of North America. In the context of this case study, this is an exclusive designation, and is not to be confused with Globally Indigenous people. I employ a Critical Indigenous lens in my analysis.

The purpose of this case study is to highlight an Indigenous experience in the school system in Canada in case study format, to provide some reflections on the experience, and to make some recommendations as to how to mitigate the experience. This will be accomplished by providing some background/ history related to the education system and Indigenous learners, a case study of PHOENIX, and asking some critical questions related to PHOENIX's experience. The questions on offer within this study are for you to use as

67

prompts for your self-reflection. I hope you will use them wisely, not on others, but on your inward journey of self-exploration.

Beginning Questions:

• What does it mean to be an Indigenous learner in school these days?
• What does racism look like?
• What does racism feel like?
• What does colonialism feel like?
• What does violence feel like?
• What does safety feel like?
• What do young Indigenous people have to put up with in order to attend school?

There are policies that have shaped the education of Indigenous children. The first is the Royal Proclamation of 1763, the next is the Gradual Civilization Act of 1857, then the Constitution Act of 1867, specifically section 91(24), the next is the Constitution Act of 1982, specifically section 35(1). As a result of federal responsibility outlined in the Indian Act of 1876, residential schools became popular as a mechanism of assimilation because they severed the relationship between child (future) and community (ancestral history). The debate of whether Indigenous people were humans or animals raged for decades among white people. While the constitution act states clearly that Indigenous people are, indeed, human, society still treats us much the way the early settlers did; like animals, and with disregard and brutality. Indigenous people are still living with the narrative of "being conquered" and it is difficult to exist in the context of always being inferior. The pervasive attitude extends well beyond racism and microaggressions. Those are gentle words to describe the experiences of Indigenous people in Canada. Case in point, from personal experience of the author: how is it that a white professor can say to an Indigenous professor "you were only hired because you are Aboriginal" and get away with it? Where does that entitlement come from? It is the colonialism that whites embody and perpetuate each day that keeps Indigenous people "in their place."

To play this out just a little bit more, I want to draw a hypothetical scenario. If an Indigenous person makes a claim to a piece of land and states clearly, and explicitly, that this is my land, the police will intervene and that person is imprisoned or shot dead in the case of Dudley George. Should I choose to walk into your house, displace you, and claim the property as my own, I will be imprisoned and you will be gently and compassionately returned to your home by authorities, all the while acknowledged in the media as a victim of violence. You will likely receive some commendation from your local mayor and some go-fund-me campaign will be created on your behalf. The argument here is that there are laws in place to protect people and to punish those who break those laws. By contrast, whites came to Turtle Island and enacted the very process noted above. The local laws were ignored, the men slaughtered, the women raped and claimed as property, and the children enslaved. Whole nations of people were intentionally murdered in a process of erasure. The first scenario is hypothetical; the second is historical fact. The white narrative is one of conquest, of victory, of seizure, of heroes defeating villains, of saints taming savages, and of historical timelines that start immediately after the great victory. Indigenous people live with the reality of what occurred before the white timeline began.

The intergenerational trauma and inherited grief and loss that each Indigenous child lives with is real. It is real because Indigenous people, as a whole, live in relative poverty, in poor conditions, in a racist society full of racist people who, after extracting and exploiting the Indigenous cultures of what is valued by whites, would rather they disappear from sight and from history.

The answer to "why didn't I learn this in school?" is one of erasure. The Statement of the Government of Canada on Indian Policy (1969 White Paper) still has teeth, and society plays out its intentions; erase treaties and the Indian Act.

In contrast to these policies, the Royal Commission on Aboriginal People (RCAP) report from 1996 outlines in remarkable depth all the ailments colonization has created for Indigenous people and the myriad ways to address the effects. The United Nations Declaration on the Rights of Indigenous Peoples (UNDRIP) from 2007 outlines for white people exactly how you should behave, but no one is forced to read it. The Truth and Reconciliation Commission (TRC) Report from 2015 offers explicit actions that are not being internalized by whites. These documents represent the best of what we have to offer, and yet they are treated as "other" by white people. It is a privilege to not have to read them. It is this privilege that perpetuates colonialism in society. It is this privilege that plays out every day against Indigenous learners in K–12 educational settings. Non-Indigenous teachers never have to consider the needs of Indigenous learners, never have to accommodate their learning styles, never have to transform themselves into the teacher that the Indigenous learner deserves. Indigenous learners are not equity seeking; they are equity deserving. All of this educating occurs on Indigenous learners' land, after all. The salaries and benefits enjoyed by non-Indigenous teachers are paid while Indigenous people starve, live in boil-water advisory conditions, die from exposure in the same communities where the non-Indigenous teachers participate in the white economy by shopping for trivial items, eat in restaurants, and enjoy leisure activities, and exercise the privilege of turning a blind eye.

We are all treaty people. What does this statement mean? It means that anyone who lives in Canada is bound by the treaties that were signed as peace agreements, also called contracts. These contracts set out rights, considerations, conditions, and payments to be made to Indigenous people, in perpetuity, in exchange for the land and its resources. Education is one of those rights. The residential school policy was one way the government fulfilled its obligation to educate Indigenous people. In the aftermath of residential schools, and the damage they created, reservation schools were created and have been a problem since their inception.

QUESTIONS

• What are the relevant Acts or policies that impact Indigenous learners?
• What is a treaty?
• What are the lasting effects of residential schools?
• What is the RCAP Report of 1996?
• What is the UNDRIP of 2007?
• What is the TRC Report of 2015?
• What are your responsibilities and obligations related to these reports?

One of the gross assumptions has always been that children on reservations achieve at lower levels when compared to their urban counterparts. I have never been witness to any sort of deconstruction of this statement. It is simply accepted as fact. So, I have been reflecting on this situation in light of this case study, and I have come to some preliminary deductions. These deductions do not rely on statistics that paint an inarticulate picture; rather, a lived experience of reservation schools and an untold truth about them. These statements cannot be captured by any research methodology because they contain a truth that people deny, for fear of judgment.

Some reservation schools are carryover institutions of residential schools. Indigenous children achieve the level of expectations. Only the most desperate of young, untrained, beginning educators accept postings at reservation schools. Many of those young teachers have some type of savior complex. The societal convention is to expect less from Indigenous learners because they are "simple, less-than, incapable, Savages, living in difficult conditions, etc." Reservation schools are underfunded, under-resourced, neglected, condemnable facilities. There are normally one or two teachers for multiple grades; often one teacher for all grades JK-8. Reservations are perceived as black holes; no one knows what goes on there, and no one cares. Funding for any activity on reservations, including education, is perceived by the public as a budgetary liability, and these perceptions exist on a continuum from favorable to damnable—those with savior complexes, with their good intentions, still regard these children as a "worthy cause." Society does not regard the education of Indigenous children as an inherent right; however, in a double-standard-sort-of-way, these same people rally against urban teachers when their own children are not taught curriculum right up to the last minute of the school year. The disparity between reservation schools and urban schools continues to grow due to malignant neglect, complacency, racism, marginalization, exclusion, and ongoing colonialism. Indigenous children are blamed for the results of all this, and society never takes the blame or responsibility. Children are the product of environment, intentions, investment, inputs, resources, ideologies, influences, subtle messages, and role modeling. The phrase "they just need to pull themselves up by the bootstraps" assumes many things, such as there is sufficient funding for boots, those boots have straps, the wearer of said boots has eaten a sufficiently nutritious and substantial meal to fuel the energy to do said pulling-up, said child has been taught the mechanics of the said action of pulling-up, said instructor role models the wearing of boots and not high-heeled shoes, and the analogy goes on and on. Standards are lower on reservation schools, but those standards are set by the provincial governments, and Band Chief-and-Council governments, like any other municipal governments, have no jurisdiction over these standards; yet, they are blamed for not prioritizing the funding or enforcing policies of the school. Do white mayors of white cities get blamed directly for what goes on in schools? The answer is no. Parents of children on reservations are blamed for not doing their part at home; yet, they are also the product of the reservation school system, colonialism, societal racism, erasure, dishonored treaties, and displacement from the land. These parents are struggling to boil sufficient water to wash and feed their families because too many Indigenous communities are on boil-water advisories. There is an assumption that there are hidden resources, whether capitalistic or innate, that magically appear. Everyone "passes the buck" and expects the next person in the line of responsibility to attend to the neglect—the best examples of which are grammar, literacy, numeracy, finances, ethics, morality, relational accountability, critical analysis, curiosity and investigation, the subtle art of deduction, and so on. You cannot teach what you do not know. Inexperienced educators burn out. What does a burned-out person have to offer? A burned-out teacher is exactly like a burned-out light bulb—they no longer shine, they offer no light to illuminate the darkness of the unknown, they still draw power from the grid (salary and benefits), and they are dangerous to the touch. Indigenous students in reservation schools normally have several teachers each year—there is no consistency or stability for these children. Ceremonies and cultural activities, such as the well-known "Goose Days" in the far north of Ontario, are not folded into the learning, the curriculum, nor are they celebrated by society.

I have heard stories from many teachers who had their "horrible" experiences up in the far north of Ontario and they all talk negatively about any activity that "interfered" with their curriculum. Teachers extract resources ($$$) from the community without ever becoming part of the community. I have heard Indigenous community members say that teachers should be mandated to participate in the community—actively engage with ceremonies, cultural activities, sit with elders, pull nets on the lake, hunt, gather medicines, participate in the preparation of community feasts. Teachers always leave for greener (urban) pastures, selfishly, leaving behind broken-hearted children who then have to grieve that loss.

CASE STORY

I am writing a narrative about PHOENIX, a gender nonspecific Indigenous person experiencing headaches at school, and night terrors at home. I will write this narrative from the perspective of a third-person observer. I am writing this case study in three parts. Drawing on your experiences, please work through the questions at the end of each part before you proceed to the next.

Part One

PHOENIX is a beautiful, dark-skinned, dark-haired, visibly Indigenous learner, in Grade 5, who has been labeled as difficult, lazy, unfortunate, and distracting by some, while also being labeled as unique, creative, expressive, interesting, enthusiastic, and sensitive by others. PHOENIX has two loving, hardworking parents who are vocal about racism in the school, and who challenge the teachers and administration to engage indigenous learners more intentionally and respectfully. PHOENIX's father is particularly vocal about the treaty rights of PHOENIX. PHOENIX has undiagnosed specific learning difficulties (SpLD) with dyslexia and dysgraphia. The parents "are doing the best they can with what they have." PHOENIX is engaged with their culture, is well read, well traveled, and has a beautiful long braid of dark hair. PHOENIX is also larger than their peers by a considerable margin.

For a brief period of approximately three weeks PHOENIX was acting out in class, claiming to have a headache every time math class started, disrupting peers, asking off-topic questions, requesting to go to the bathroom frequently, and generally presenting distracted behavior. This behavior was communicated home to PHOENIX's parents who said they would talk with PHOENIX. When asked what is going on, and what is causing your headaches and distraction at school, PHOENIX shared that math gives them a headache. A discourse about how the world is unsafe started to permeate dinner conversation. Furthermore, the discourse included questions and bold statements about "mean people" and "evil people," and about vengeance. Lastly, as a talented visual artist, PHOENIX's sketches started to take on darker themes of violence, death, blood, and fire. The themes of conversation, and drawing, were well out of character for PHOENIX. This concerned the parents, especially given PHOENIX's gender identity. PHOENIX's parents began to wonder if PHOENIX had entered a "dark period" or if it was hormonal, or if there was an external cause to the change of nature and demeanor.

Drawing on your experiences and training, please answer the following questions:

1. What are your assumptions and biases about PHOENIX?
2. What are your assumptions and biases about the parents?
3. What are your instincts and intuition telling you about this situation?
4. What is your formulation of a solution at this point in the case study?

Part Two

Soon thereafter, PHOENIX entered the schoolyard with their father before school, and was excited to play with friends from their class. The school bell rang and PHOENIX lined up to enter school. PHOENIX's father departed. The school day progressed without incident until after the first break. PHOENIX's father was called to the school to pick up PHOENIX because they hit, and injured, another child in the schoolyard during the break. Upon arrival, PHOENIX's father asked them what happened, but PHOENIX refused to answer. The father asked the principal and vice-principal what happened. The father was told that PHOENIX grabbed another child and punched them. The father asked if PHOENIX was provoked and was told that they were not. This occurred on four separate occasions over the course of two weeks. The father became angry and aggressive with the teachers and administration at the school, threatening to take legal action for their neglectful treatment of PHOENIX. The parents used words such as racism, sexism, and called for an inquiry.

QUESTIONS

1. What are your assumptions and biases about PHOENIX?
2. What are your assumptions and biases about the parents?
3. What are your instincts and intuition telling you about this situation?
4. What is your formulation of a solution at this point in the case study?

Part Three

PHOENIX's father informed the principal of the school that he would be
attending school for the day to observe PHOENIX throughout the day. After
a period of argument over disrupting the flow of the school day, making
children feel uncomfortable, and concerns over what other parents might say,
the principal relented/consented. The father observed that the game of choice
on each break was "tag." Inevitably, PHOENIX wound up being "it" during
the game, and for extended periods of time. This would frustrate PHOENIX
and they would ask the other children to change games, repeatedly. The
other children would eventually allow PHOENIX to tag out, but within two
tags among a group of twelve children, PHOENIX would end up being "it"
again; a respite of approximately 1 minute. The game turned ugly as each of
the other kids would run circles around PHOENIX, while keeping just out of
reach, and pull hard on their braid of hair while making "INDIAN" noises
while patting their mouths with their hands. This made PHOENIX visibly
angry until PHOENIX was lying on the ground holding their head from a
headache, caused by all the hairpulling, and crying. The father intervened
before PHOENIX could retaliate again and withdrew PHOENIX from school
until such a time that the principal met with the parents of the other children.
The father declared that there were acts of bullying and racism occurring in
the schoolyard right in front of teachers on duty, all under the leadership of the
school administrators. The father asked PHOENIX why they bother playing
with those children at all, and the answer was that they liked the other children, and indeed one of the children was their best friend. The father insisted
that the situation be dealt with immediately and in comprehensive fashion.

QUESTIONS

1. How accurate were your assumptions and biases about PHOENIX?
2. How accurate were your assumptions and biases about the parents?
3. Did your instincts and intuition about the situation impair your ability to
   attend to PHOENIX?
4. Was your formulation of a solution helpful?
5. Why was PHOENIX experiencing headaches?
6. Why was PHOENIX protecting the "best friend"?
7. What is the correct course of action in this situation?
8. What is your role in supporting PHOENIX in this situation?
9. What is your role in addressing the bullying?
10. What are some of the signs of racism, sexism, ableism, and bullying that
    you should be looking for, all the time?
11. What can you do to be more situationally aware as an educator?

TAKEAWAYS

The risk here is to focus on the labels of dyslexia and dysgraphia, the difficult parents, the disruptive behavior of the student, and the innocent play of the classmates. This would be a mistake. The lens to use here is one of systemic racism, heteronormativity, ableism, sexism, and moreover, colonialism.

How does the section on reservation schools relate to PHOENIX? This Indigenous student is the product of generations of Indigenous people who have gone through reservation schooling, residential schooling and who have experienced all of what was stated in the above paragraph. It is the context in which PHOENIX has been raised, and the worldview that permeates this young person's life. Simply put, it is an intergenerational truth of First Nations, rural, and urban Indigenous people who have survived the white school system. There is trauma attached to education for Indigenous people, regardless of what they might say to your face.

RECOMMENDATIONS

1. Read the RCAP report from 1996: https://publications.gc.ca/Collection -R/LoPBdP/EB/prb9924-e.htm
2. Read the Truth and Reconciliation report from 2015: https://www.rcaanc -cirnac.gc.ca/eng/1450124405592/1529106060525
3. Read the UNDRIP from 2007: https://www.un.org/development/desa/ indigenouspeoples/declaration-on-the-rights-of-indigenous-peoples.html
4. Read the Constitution Act sections 91(24) and 35(1): https://laws-lois .justice.gc.ca/eng/Const/index.html
5. Read the White Paper from 1969: https://indigenousfoundations.arts.ubc .ca/the_white_paper_1969/
6. Read about Indigenous wholism (see Hill, 2021): https://www.jcharlton- publishing.com/product/indigenous-healing-voices-of-elders-and-healers/
7. Engage relational accountability in teaching: https://scholars.wlu.ca/cgi /viewcontent.cgi?referer=https://www.google.com/&httpsredir=1&arti- cle=1014&context=scwk_faculty

CONCLUSION AND CRITICAL QUESTIONING

While you may never "know" what it is like to be an Indigenous learner, like PHOENIX, you can engage in critical self-reflection to further your capacity for ethical relational engagement. You need to develop greater awareness of contextual factors that may not be readily apparent. Each child is an ecosystem, and each of those ecosystems interacts with one another. You are also an ecosystem, and this requires careful consideration as you engage Indigenous children because the inherent biases, assumptions, values, beliefs, and world-views of different ecosystems can cause trespasses, transgressions, wounding, and violations. What does it mean to be white? This is not just about deconstructing white privilege, or how you benefit from ongoing colonialism, or class analysis, but also about what values, beliefs, biases, assumptions, and reflexes you embody. Good educators examine their own worldviews and work to mitigate the potential negative impacts of their worldviews on children that have been raised in different worldviews. This is a lesson in diversity.

While it is absolutely critical to engage in a learning journey about the cultures of the Indigenous children in your care, it is nearly equally important to not put those children on the spot with a "trivia Q&A" to demonstrate just how much you think you know. While well-intentioned and relational, the Q&A sessions create great discomfort for Indigenous learners. What can you do? You can learn and then integrate the "knowledge" into your way of seeing, being, knowing, and doing. This type of cultural learning is for you to develop an awareness, but not an expertise; it is about self-reflection on your own epistemology, rather than an external expression of perceived understanding or knowing. It is critical to understand that just because you read something, hear something, or watch something, does not mean you "know" about something. Indigenous cultures represent what I call embodied knowledge, and the embodiment is not a passing fancy; it is a way of seeing, being, knowing, and doing. What does this look like in practice? A teacher who is truly engaged with Indigenous students might ask the question "Have you ever heard of X-cultural-piece-of-knowledge?" If the student says yes, it could be a sharing opportunity, and possibly a relationship-building moment. If the student says no, it could be an opportunity to ask if they would like to learn about it together. Much information about Indigenous cultures is written, and much is on display with some regularity throughout the year.

What is the experience of Indigenous learners in grade school? Indigenous people have always been outsiders in the education system, coming from different worldviews, and have been treated in forcefully assimilative ways. The education system does not recognize or celebrate difference and is constructed to reinforce colonial rule of this land. Indigenous students are evaluated against criteria that are foreign, are forced to sit all day in rows, to raise their hands in a competitive way to be heard or are called on out-of-the-blue to answer questions. One simple strategy is to construct a classroom as a circle and to use a talking stick so that every student understands that it is their turn to answer a question when the talking stick comes to them and that they are not to speak when they are not holding the talking stick. This is a more inclusive and equitable facilitation process.

What are the needed resources to help Indigenous students succeed? One way to support Indigenous students is to start with safety. It is not safe to ask an Indigenous student to raise their hand and compete with others to be heard. It is, likewise, not safe to call on them randomly. Using circle process is simple and effective for all learners. It inherently quashes competition. It creates predictable engagement. Some very obvious strategies are to use inclusive resources such as audio, video, and textual materials that represent the diversity of cultures within the learning group. Additionally, guests from cultural groups who can speak about experiences of culture can be very impactful. As an Indigenous learner, I recall very few exceptionally great days in K–12 school; however, the most memorable day was when one of my elders from my community was invited to spend the day at my school. As soon as we saw each other we hugged, and he spoke to me in our language. He made some jokes and I was laughing, and he asked if I could be his helper for the day. He was a family friend, and one of my ceremonial elders, and his presence at my school for that one day buoyed my spirit for weeks to come. I was more focused and productive because I was supported, and I felt that the school was a safe place where elders occasionally visited.

What can you do in your everyday life to transform yourself into a relational being? What can you do to go out of your way to make PHOENIX's life at school safe? What is your role, and in what ways are you complicit, in the racism, discrimination, and bullying experienced by PHOENIX? You are a treaty person. You benefit directly from the treaties signed by your ancestors. In what ways are you, personally, going to honor the treaties from which you benefit on a daily basis? It is your responsibility to be a good relation to Indigenous people. As an educator you are an instrument of the treaties that promise education to Indigenous people.

It is a well-known fact that curriculum does not reflect the knowledge systems of Indigenous people. It is a well-known fact that the popular pedagogy used in the current grade school curriculum does not capture the majority of learning styles. It is a well-known fact that there are greater numbers of students with SpLD than meet the eye.

These are structural deficits in the K–12 education system that negatively impact the majority of learners. The marginalization this creates for Indigenous learners is compounded exponentially.

I propose educating from the margins. I propose a pedagogy of universal design that attends to every learner's wholistic development. I compel teachers to engage in wholistic assessment of learners. I promote "seeing" and "knowing" your students. Treat them like family and community. Build a trusting, mutual relationship, and then take intentional steps to not betray that trust. The relationship is the vehicle in which intention travels toward action. The intention is student success. The action is doing what it takes to ensure the successful outcome for each student. I do not approve of activities such as assessment for the purpose of punitive action. What does punitive action look like? Referrals to child protection, reports to police, reports to welfare workers, and so on. I encourage teachers to untrain themselves in ways that are judgmental, biased toward a single way of teaching and learning, toxically white, and singular.

Miigwetch, All My Relations.

REFERENCES

Dussault, R., & Erasmus, G. (1996). *Report of the royal commission on Aboriginal Peoples*. https://publications.gc.ca/Collection-R/LoPBdP/EB/prb9924-e.htm.

Hill, G. (2021). *Indigenous healing: Voices of elders and healers*. JCharlton Press Inc.

Truth and Reconciliation Commission of Canada. (2015). *Honouring the truth, reconciling for the future: Summary of the final report of the truth and reconciliation commission of Canada*. https://www.rcaanc-cirnac.gc.ca/eng/1450124405592/1529106060525.

Section 2

INTERMEDIATE/HIGH SCHOOL (7–12) SECTION OVERVIEW

Mental health concerns can persist into the intermediate and high school years and beyond or can newly emerge within adolescence well into adulthood. In this section, we are first introduced to a seventeen-year-old (Maia) in New Zealand who is struggling with the social transition to a physically distant tertiary school setting (Case Story #8: Building a Community of Care in New Zealand: To what question is exclusion ever the answer? contributors Christina Belcher and Kimberly Maich). In this case, exclusion and loneliness were remediated with a community of care approach to support this enthusiastic but overextended student. Case Story #9 is entitled (Re)framing Mental Health in Argentina (contributor Javier Alejandro Rojas). This case takes us through the case of twelve-year-old Lautaro who was faced with conflicts between family expectations and school demands complicated by his need for emotional and cognitive self-regulation skill-building. We are then made aware of the Medical Model of Mental Health in Iran (Case Story #10; contributor Tayebeh Sohrabi) through the case of Grade-7 student Sarah, where Sarah and her family are struggling to find available services in a specialized school setting following disability-based exclusion from the public school system. Case Story #11 (How to strengthen a child's vulnerability by providing support at school? Case study from Croatia; contributors Sanja Skočić Mihić, Zorica Janković, Sanja Tatalović Vorkapić, and Snježana Sekušak Galešev) shares with us the narrative of Marko, a fifteen-year-old student with a developmental disability and behavior and emotional issues, but from the point of view of a psychotherapist in school-based practice. As a vulnerable adolescent, Marko experienced social isolation, exclusion, bullying, and aggression at school. In Case Story #12 (Trauma and School Supports in the United States; contributors Erika Brindopke and Meaghan McCollow), we learn about Iosefina, a Grade-10 student, with a specific learning disability, trauma, and emotional issues, necessitating placement in a counseling-rich classroom program. This narrative is from the point of view of the school's mental health counselor. Lastly, we introduce Jean-Pierre, a seventeen-year-old from Haiti in Case Story #13 (Despite the Best of Intentions: A Case of Mental Health in a Fragile Context in Haiti; contributors: Steve Sider and Samuel Charles) whose family was displaced from their home due to a recent earthquake and forced to move to a new city to attend high school under precarious environmental and economic conditions. Maia, Lautaro, Sarah, Mark, Iosfina, and Jean-Pierre all help us learn about the challenges of reaching and teaching students with complex mental health needs in the adolescent years.

Chapter 8

Case Story #8—Building a Community of Care in New Zealand

To what question is exclusion ever the answer?

Christina Belcher and Kimberly Maich

It is February, and the school year is beginning again in New Zealand. I am currently teaching in a tertiary institution, which is any institution offering educational degrees beyond Grade 11 in New Zealand. As my tertiary students introduce themselves, I am captivated by a young seventeen-year-old from one of our Oceania islands. (In New Zealand, the word "university" is protected by law. There are six universities and there shall be no more. A *tertiary institute* is one that offers post-K–12 education at the university level on the New Zealand Qualifications Framework which governs educational facilities including teaching qualifications.) I have rarely seen a student so enthusiastic about being in class on the first day—even though she was far from home.

Sending money back to the islands is very common for Pasifika peoples: the name of people living on the independent islands surrounding New Zealand. Family and church come first. These reasons are often why young people come to New Zealand in the first place: to be able to support their family at home, such as school fees for siblings and money for church upkeep. They are taught to think of others before themselves. Culturally, the desire to serve is paramount. But on the other hand, there are built-in expectations which have also developed into part of the culture. If there is a big celebration, such as a coronation, each village is required to provide something—and they will have to do their bit for that. Maia is here with a goal of eventually being the first certified teacher when she returns to her island. She is warmly received by her peers and settles in well.

However, as the weeks go by, I notice that Maia is not as effervescent. She does not appear to stop for morning tea or lunch and often rushes off the minute the last class of the day ends. She looks tired and stressed but is still doing very good work on her assignments. Her peers are concerned and are asking me about her, so I make it my business to intercept her between class and morning tea, confidentially, to see how she is doing.

As we chat, I discover that part of Maia's family culture is that every child in the family must pay one bill per month to support the parents and home on the island, reflecting Pasifika values. Maia is expected to pay a very large bill, because being off the island she makes more money than her siblings do on the island. Therefore, Maia has taken on cleaning for an elderly aunt every Saturday, shopping and cooking for an uncle every weekday evening, and babysitting two children for a cousin and her husband who are on shift work between 6:00 am and 8:00 am every weekday morning. Her chores for them were getting the children fed and ready for school between the hours when her husband left for his shift at 6:00 am and her aunt returned at 8:00 am. Maia then comes directly to her class and courses. Maia also makes and sells crafts at the Sunday community market twice a month. On top of it all, Maia said she was feeling lonely and homesick. She wanted to be with her peers—but could not manage the time or energy.

This situation was a problem.

Maia did not want to feel excluded from her new social family of peers and social school experiences but had very little extra time and energy to socialize during the day. Other students were misunderstanding her apologies for not attending as disinterest in accepting their invitations. Since we all meet daily as a class in a common room and share lunch, her peers soon became aware of her predicament—by invitation of Maia—who seemed to be relieved to be able to tell them about the stresses of her current situation that were impacting her mental health and sense of well-being. Although Maia is clearly able to handle stress well, and she has shared that she just gets on with it, it was obvious that she was struggling to maintain the balance between work and school with only herself to rely on through the tough times.

So, what could we, as a community of learners and future educators, do? There were options. We could try to assist Maia by crafting one extra product a week for the market and donate earned funds if we had talents in this area, but that takes time away from personal study, and this kind of help may not be appropriate to her culture. We could make cards of encouragement, but this may ebb after a week or so. We could perhaps engage in a fundraising event, but that may be embarrassing. These were all suggested to me by Maia's peers in our endeavor to be a supportive community, but they all had some shortcomings and no secure participant accountability.

In the end, we decided together to initiate pot luck lunches every school day during our communal lunchtime and become a surrogate community. This would mean a change in most of our personal daily schedules. It necessitated moving our main meals to lunch and our lighter meals to the end of the day. Since most of my students did not live with their families, this change was not a problem for them. We all took turns in teams of five (there were twenty of us, including myself), bringing the meal, so each team was responsible for contributing some element of a meal about once a week. We all picked one day for consistency—Friday. We made daily menus. Some teams decided to cook traditional food. Some opted to do a barbecue. Others opted for pizza or fish and chips to be brought in as take out once a week.

To what question is exclusion ever the answer? In deciding that, to no question is exclusion and loneliness ever the answer, this collaborative community venture resulted in some of the best memories we ever made—and better support systems and mental wellness for many, including the overextended Maia.

BRIEF CRITICAL RESPONSE QUESTIONS

1. Is there a definition of mental health specific to New Zealand? If so, what is it? If not, why not?
2. What does extended family mean to you? How does your experience compare to Maia's?
3. What might have happened to Maia if her peers had not cared about her well-being?
4. What might have happened to Maia if her tertiary teacher had not cared about her well-being?
5. Why is peer support significant to mental health—at any age?

REFLECTIVE RESPONSE QUESTIONS

1. How might this situation have played out if the involved educator had not attended to the local cultural demands of Maia's life?
2. What lessons can be learned about creating a supportive and collaborative community for peer-to-peer mental health support?
3. Less seems to be written about support services in higher education. Why would this be the case?
4. Should Maia be trying to balance her own personal mental health needs with the demands of her extended family? Why or why not?
5. Do we tend to set aside adolescent issues as normative struggles which are to be expected? Why or why not?

POSSIBLE SUPPORT STRATEGIES

- Consistency in peer-to-peer social contact
- Informal peer check-ins for mental health status
- Psychoeducational counseling with a boundary-setting focus
- Acceptance and understanding of cultural diversity

CONCLUSION

- Observing the observed deterioration of mental health in a teaching and learning environment (tied to Cushman et al., 2011; Denny et al., 2018)
- Acting upon the observed deterioration of mental health while considering privacy and confidentiality (tied to Cushman et al., 2011; Denny et al., 2018)
- The necessity of a supportive peer community during adolescent sturm und drang (tied to Johns, 2017)
- The role of healthy eating in relation to positive mental health (tied to Kulkarni et al., 2012)
- The role of ongoing, sustained support if formal mental health interventions are uninvited, misunderstood, or unwelcome (tied to the work of Mariu et al., 2012—see references)

LINKS

- Mental Health Foundation of New Zealand: https://www.mentalhealth.org.nz/get-help/a-z/resource/14/depression-youth
- Ministry of Health: https://www.health.govt.nz/nz-health-statistics/health-statistics-and-data-setds/child-and-youth-health-data-and-stats
- New Zealand Qualifications Authority: https://www.nzqa.govt.nz/nqfdocs/units/pdf/27461.pdf
- New Zealand Qualifications Authority, Mental Health & Addictions: https://www.nzqa.govt.nz/nqfdocs/units/pdf/26985.pdf
- New Zealand Qualifications Authority Tertiary Education: https://www.nzqa.govt.nz/studying-in-new-zealand/tertiary-education/ Pasifika Values: https://www.massey.ac.nz/massey/students/pasifika-student-services/staff-resources/values.cfm
- Community & Public Health: https://www.cph.co.nz/your-health/youth-mental-health/
- Government of New Zealand, Well-being at Home & School: https://parents.education.govt.nz/secondary-school/wellbeing/mental-health/

- School & Mental Health: A Student Perspective (Education Central): https://educationcentral.co.nz/school-and-mental-health-a-student-per-spective/?fbclid=IwAR17nGEwrlPOQbPcnQx01_FxdBagOsa0ZZv5U SI6OrLVEvIxuWrdTqWEzw Teachers Must Step in on Mental Health (Newsroom): https://www.newsroom.co.nz/2018/07/15/152033/schools -must-cater-to-mental-health-needs?fbclid=IwAR14laH4272TngMgJdIZQ WUSKtb8XYrYivBkfC9pDcuGKfwgjhx4WoTg8EM

REFERENCES

Cushman, P., Clelland, T., & Hornby, G. (2011). Health-promoting schools and mental health issues: A survey of New Zealand schools. *Pastoral Care in Education: International Associate Editors*, *29*(4), 247–260. https://doi.org/10.1080/02643944 .2011.626066.

Denny, S., Howie, H., Grant, S., Galbreath, R., Utter, J., Fleming, T., & Clark, T. (2018). Characteristics of school-based health services associated with students' mental health. *Journal of Health Services Research & Policy*, *23*(1), 7–14. https:// doi.org/10.1177/1355819617716196.

Johns, C. (2017). Mental health and wellbeing in New Zealand education. *Journal of Initial Teacher Inquiry*, *3*, 61–54. https://ir.canterbury.ac.nz/handle/10092/14629.

Kulkarni, A., Swinburn, B., & Utter, J. (2015). Associations between diet quality and mental health in socially disadvantaged New Zealand adolescents. *European Journal of Clinical Nutrition*, *69*(1), 79–83. https://doi.org/10.1038/ejcn.2014.130.

Mariu, K., Merry, S., Robinson, E., & Watson, P. (2012). Seeking professional help for mental health problems, among New Zealand secondary school students. *Clinical Child Psychology and Psychiatry*, *17*(2), 284–297. https://doi.org/10.1177 /1359104511404176.

Chapter 9

Case Story #9—(Re)framing Mental Health in Argentina

Javier Alejandro Rojas

THEORETICAL MODEL AND BACKGROUND

Lautaro is a twelve-year-old boy in Grade 7 of the Argentinian primary school who is hoping to advance next year to secondary school. The case of Lautaro applies the psychological theory of cognition and behavior considering a comprehensive and inclusive intervention perspective that involves active roles for Lautaro, his family, school staff, and school integration support team and external mental health professionals assigned by social insurance plans. Mental health practice in Argentinian school—which is available only for a few people who are able to access such services—is based on a comprehensive assessment of the student's required social, communication, and learning skills to overcome successfully their daily challenges in school. Such an intervention model reinforces Lautaro's habits and daily routines in authentic school activities and is oriented to model cognition and behavior in a joint effort of family, school, and mental health supports to prevent him from reacting to his most common anxiety triggers.

The music therapist, psychologist, and school integration team agree to compliment intervention activities in school, home, and psychotherapy sessions to treat his persistent nonstop death-themed narrative. Lautaro uses this narrative to interrupt class lessons and focus the attention of everyone around him on death issues like it is an entertaining topic to emphasize all day long. During class lessons, he quotes people's deaths portrayed in documentaries, urban legends, television shows, books, and video games that he enjoys at home. Some teachers state that his death-themed obsession has also been influenced by his grief process of his recent father's departure and her mother's belief that Lautaro must take his father's male role to lead their home and give her and his two younger brothers emotional security.

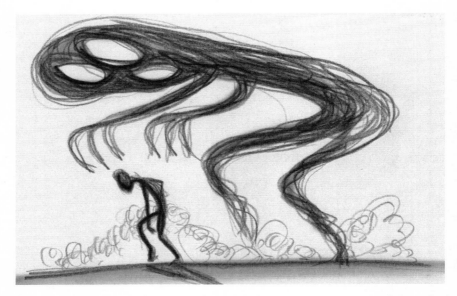

Figure 9.1   When art tells a story about emotion. Case Story #9. *iStock—Standard License.* https://stock.adobe.com/ca/images/depression-and-sadness-concept-artwork /158584607?prev_url=detail.

Lautaro's mother has become angry each time the school staff demands a commitment to making sure Lautaro comes to school on time every day. Although she has been assigned mental health professionals for supporting two younger Lautaro's brothers in both school and home, she typically responds that they are running late because she has to struggle daily for parenting her three sick children alone. She refers to *sick children* because the Argentinian mental health system in school is accessible only through school support for students who are able to apply and qualify for a disability certificate approved by a medical board, which are managed by social insurance plans. Likewise, external professionals that offer such mental health support in school are hired by nonprofit organizations (NGOs) that manage school integration programs funded by social insurance plans. Only a few students are able to use mental health services in Argentinian schools if their families or families' employers pay a social insurance plan and if they fall under eligibility criteria to apply for a disability certificate. Fortunately, Lautaro has been assigned such mental health support not only weekly through music therapy and psychotherapy sessions but also through an NGO-based mental health professional to support him in some of their school activities.

Lautaro's mother has had several conflicts with the school staff because she argues that Lautaro is not able to join his classmates' camping trip, which would mean temporarily leaving his family where he is now in his father's role, which is unacceptable. According to the school staff and external mental health professionals who treat Lautaro, she wields such an argument to prevent him from a significant social experience in which their classmates will celebrate their primary school graduation before his secondary school entry. In particular, Lautaro and the external mental health professionals who treat him advise her mother to begin a psychotherapeutic treatment not only for coping with his husband's recent demise but also for changing her perception of Lautaro's role. She acknowledges her necessity for psychotherapeutic support and agrees to begin this treatment as soon as possible.

Although Lautaro is always late for school, he is not able to hang out sometimes with his classmates outside school due to his family's claims on his time, and has daily conflicts with his teachers because of his nonstop death-themed narrative during class lessons, he loves to spend time at school. However, this background has influenced other anxiety and low self-confidence triggers that come up in daily school activities making him go through difficult situations in school regarding his grades and failed courses.

LAUTARO'S STORY

I am waiting for Lautaro at the school's front desk to accompany him to his classroom. He is running late as usual. His teacher does not usually begin any class lesson before he arrives at his classroom since he always becomes anxious, cries, and cannot stop interrupting his classmates and teachers by talking about how missing even a tiny bit of a class lesson will cause him to fail such course. However, it is 8:20 already and she has decided to begin today's lesson class without him. When I am about to send a message to his mother to ask what happened and if he would come today to school, Lautaro slams the main school door and runs quickly through the first-floor hall and then upstairs toward his classroom.

As soon as I arrive at his classroom door, I find his teacher yelling at him because he had slammed the classroom door without asking for permission to enter and interrupted a classmate's presentation. He ignores his teacher and persists, instead, in asking what he missed and if such a missed lesson will be essential to be able to answer the next exam questions. Although his teacher responds several times in a calming way, Lautaro yells at her that it will fail his exams. His teacher, classmates, and a mental health professional try unsuccessfully to calm him down without excluding him from his classroom but eventually his teacher asks him to leave. Lautaro is devastated and begins to cry, yell, run around the school halls, and slap his hands on the other teachers' doors until his teacher allows him to come back to her classroom space.

During his next class lesson, Lautaro feels less nervous, anxious, and angry because there he can demonstrate his outstanding knowledge, analysis, and memory abilities to discuss complex topics with his teacher which helps him to stand out above his classmates. However, his anxiety triggers arise again when he has to find specific information in his course notebook. He struggles to find it immediately due to his usual messy notes. He raises his voice again, crying and yelling out that he will not be able to find the solution. Then he throws his notebook sheets out around the classroom floor. His classmates try to help him to find the notebook page he needs while he hits his head and desk with his fists. His teacher and classmates look at each other without having any clue about what more they could do to help him to overcome this particular challenge. Lautaro's problem behavior is increasing in frequency and intensity.

When his teacher hands him out his last exam grade, he is quite confident that his grade will be better than all of his classmates' grades since he had been asking them about their exam grades to highlight that he is the smartest student. He tells them that he does not need to complete homework to have good grades. He states that he prefers to invest all his mother's money buying the most recently released video games and spend all his time playing them or watching war and death-themed movies and documentaries. In fact, his narrative that constantly interrupt his teachers and classmates during classes is based on talking nonstop about such topics—when he is not talking about death. Some of his classmates ask why he prefers to buy video games instead of buying school supplies since they have noticed that he is short on such supplies, yet another source of anxiety for Lautaro. When it is his turn to be notified about his exam grade, his teacher hands it out to Lautaro. He reacts by yelling at her why he has failed this exam. She responds to him that he always rushes to give it back first to feel the smartest but instead he misunderstands the exam questions and overlooks a lot of details. He begins to cry and breaks his pencils and notebooks, and clothes. Lautaro rips up, wrinkles, and throws the exam paper at the teacher since she does not want to allow him to take it again now that he was told which questions he answered wrong. He states that he is stupid, and he never will pass primary school because he only deserves to be classified as mentally retarded.

As support settings, the school staff, external school integration support, and health professionals have designed join intervention strategies and resources according to his particular necessities for mental health support. Such intervention tools have been oriented not only to support him but also to adjust his teachers' expectations by guiding them step by step regarding his updated school integration goals according to their teaching styles. Some teachers have implemented gamification settings based on inclusive and responsive group learning support.

Supports for Lautaro are focused on improving his emotional and cognitive self-regulation skills by taking advantage of his high engagement to play video games, outstanding memory abilities, and well-developed analytic skills. Thus, he is assigned a leadership role to teach and guide his classmates within a cooperative curricular knowledge game training his empathy skills to increase the time he waits for his turn to talk while he hears his classmates' class presentations and learns from their mistakes. These self-regulation skills scaffold him to learn from procedures more than from instant results while gaining self-confidence and autonomy required to learn from his mistakes and enjoy his particular learning process. Gamification-based supports also prevents anxiety triggers linked to a lack of resilience skills from coming up when he fails exams and his flexible thinking does not make him able to take risks for changing his habitual methods to solve problems that require new methods and other strategic planning during an exam or classwork.

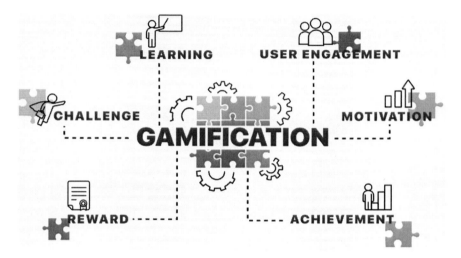

Figure 9.2   Benefits of gamilification. Case Story #9. *iStock—Standard License.* https://stock.adobe.com/ca/images/gamification-concept-infographics-chart-with-keywords-and-icons-vector-illustration/404263185?prev_url=detail.

Other teachers have implemented support such as making Lautaro spend time out of the classroom or write down some stories in a notebook based on his persistent death-themed thoughts to decrease his nonstop narrative and increase his emotional and behavioral self-regulation. Firm instructions during class lessons and workshops based on his daily classwork have been oriented to encourage him to follow step-by-step instructions focusing on processes and attention to detail more than instant results or good grades. Scheduling for school and home such as playing video games only in a specific frame time and controlled way, taking care of diet and sleep times, committing to his homework and classwork, and other habits that will improve school performance without involving any anxiety trigger are emphasized. Performing a role in a theater play where there is not a grade to evaluate school performance may also be helpful for Lautaro to get to a place of improvement, functioning, and success.

BRIEF CRITICAL RESPONSE QUESTIONS

1. Discuss with other teachers and school staff which social, emotional, and cognitive skills you should take into account to implement your curriculum plan in order to promote his self-regulation habits through daily school activities.
2. How might you face school situations in which he has failed exams or obtained low grades by teaching him coping mechanisms, reorient his adrenaline triggers, and thus to prevent him from usual anxiety triggers?
3. Browse through online examples regarding gamification activities and tools you could use for scaffolding him helped by his classmates regarding his schooling commitment, self-confidence, and autonomy to solve by himself classwork and homework for only practice purposes without any exam or grade involved.
4. Perform a literature search for gamification articles that demonstrate empirically both effective learning and higher students' engagement results to focus on class presentations by using specific classroom strategies, audiovisual and technology resources that you could adapt to enhance his attention to detail during class presentations, increase his waiting periods to talk and learn from his classmate's mistakes and teachers' explanations. Explain why these adjustments of the class lesson would modify the difficulty or make presentations more appealing to prevent students from get boring or lose their attention when more dense concepts are explained.
5. Review handbooks and other computational thinking literature that show a few examples about how to help students focus on attention to detail by investing enough time that allows them to follow your own pace in a learning activity to figure out patterns from required procedures to solve challenging problems which cannot be solved by old methods and usual tools.
6. Browse through online examples about how he could build his leadership by working in team projects, developing assertive relationships with his classmates, and gaining self-confidence to take care of himself and others without assuming social roles that belong to other people through role performance either in a theater play or workshops oriented to learn cooperatively curricular contents.

REFLECTIVE RESPONSE QUESTIONS

1. Lautaro's technology teacher gives him a leadership role to guide his classmates in order to build a clepsydra as a team. However, he comes late to class and forgot the materials required to build it. Considering that he usually starts to cry and anxiously destroys his clothes when he is excluded from school activities or has a high risk to fail grades, what do you do to teach him to assume commitment and responsibility in school activities? Also, reflecting on the school culture in Canada, why do you think that such teaching action will prevent him from repeating the same behavior in similar situations in future?

2. Examining the parenting practices and the kind of relationships built between school and family in Canada, how do you explain to Lautaro why his mother told him that if he decides to join his classmates for camp travel, when he comes back, she and his brothers will be dead? What supporting resources would you use to support your arguments, enhance his empathy skills to understand his mother's actions and coping mechanisms required to be autonomous with his final decision?

3. Name, describe, and explain three other elements you would add to Lautaro's support program in order to increase his cognitive and emotional self-regulation to be able to identify relevant information or patterns and follow his own pace to solve new step-by-step problems during exams. Explain why you would choose such elements by supporting your arguments on peer-reviewed literature.

4. Name, describe, and explain one or two elements you would remove from Lautaro's support program to prevent him from talking nonstop about war, death, money, videogames, or other interesting topics for him but not related to the class lessons subject. Support your choices to argue about why they are not useful to orient his empathy and class participation assertively.

5. Which strategy you would use to articulate and implement a comprehensive supporting plan with some teachers and school staff that do not like to teach guided by an inclusive model which considers the classmates' different ways of learning, motivations, needs, and interests? Would you prefer to work alone or persist to work jointly with the school staff? How would you work with the school staff, family, and mental health professionals taking advantage of the regulatory Canadian procedures for mental health in school? Why do you choose that option and why this choice will have better results in the mid- and long term as support strategy?

STRATEGIES OF SUPPORT TO CONSIDER

1. Objects that allow him to channel his anger or anxiety through their perceived affordances (i.e., texture, shape, color, material, size, symbolic representation attributes) when stressful situations come up.
2. Visual support as a concrete model to repeat multiple times new procedures and learn their patterns; figure out his own abstract methods to be generalized and solve similar problems; focus on step-by-step procedures of problems in which the solutions are provided in advance.
3. Behavior-tracking notebook to collect actions and attitudes by describing school activities in detail, learning goals, their elements interacting, and dynamics used.
4. Shared notebook with family to make mutual feedback about conflict situations in school or at home that could affect his emotional self-regulation and self-confidence skills to be autonomous and solve step-by-step classwork and homework (e.g., large food intakes as an anxiety response; effects of poor sleep, feeling hunger, or compulsive intake of energy drinks or caffeinated beverages; reinforcement of low self-esteem perceptions; daily conflicts with relatives).
5. List of relaxing activities, supporting strategies, and ludic tools to be used according to different conflict situations by implementing them instantly through easily identifiable and mnemonic visual aids such as pictures, short phrases, drawings, and charts.
6. Allocate shelves in school to promote his habits for preparing school supplies in advance.
7. Ask him for folders labeled with colors to support his emotional self-regulation and cognitive planning skills by organizing his notes taken in class through easily identifiable notebook marks.

CONCLUSION

- Based on gamification empirical research findings in classrooms, discuss how gamification as a how-to-do training strategy oriented to teachers could be applied as a set of behavior reinforcement resources to daily school non-gamification activities.
- As validated by some research findings of comprehensive and inclusive education curriculum in the classroom, discuss how to support his school transition from primary to secondary school by taking into account the articulation between the external mental health professionals, school staff, and family support.

- Ties to peer-reviewed articles regarding effective training of self-regulation, metacognition, and assertiveness skills under classroom management goals and consensual rules for the classroom interaction.
- Ties to literature to train attention to detail and tidiness through instructions for whole class and adjustment of explicit one-to-one-based instructions.
- Ties to literature about how to understand anxiety triggers and teach coping strategies in the classroom.
  - Mental Health Classroom Resource: https://smh-assist.ca/emhc/
  - Classroom mental health: https://classroommentalhealth.org/
  - Teacher Resources: https://cmho.org/teacher-resources/
  - Mental Health Online Resources for Educators: https://more.hmhc.ca/

LINKS TO RELEVANT ONLINE MATERIALS/VIDEOS

- Mentally Healthy Schools and Classrooms: https://smho-smso.ca/educators/learn-more/explore-by-topic/mentally-healthy-classrooms/
- The Fifteen Best Gamification Resources for Trainers and Educators: https://blog.capterra.com/15-best-gamification-resources-trainers-educators/
- Gamification is key to nudging collective behaviour | Kerstin Oberprieler | TEDxCanberra: https://youtu.be/R6F0CuzEu0A
- Mental Health and Gamification—Our Gamified World: https://youtu.be/fit_cf65FGw
- Computational Thinking: What Is It? How Is It Used?: https://youtu.be/qbnTZCj0ugI
- Computational Thinking: https://youtu.be/K3vwRQCfTHc

Chapter 10

Case Story #10—Medical Model of Mental Health in Iran

Tayebeh Sohrabi

Exceptional children in the Iranian educational system are those children who need special education services and extensive support to use their full potential. They need educational services because they differ in one or more of the following categories: They may have mental disabilities, learning disabilities, emotional disturbances, physical disabilities, speech and language disorders, hearing or visual impairments, or in contrast they can be outstanding and talented (Exceptional Children Education Organization, 2020). The Iranian Special Education Organization (ISEO) has accepted the Grossman (1983) definition of intellectual disability and divides this group of people into three categories: educable, trainable, and custodial. ISEO is responsible for the education and training of the educable students (Ministry of Education, ISEO definitions section, quoted in Bigdeli, 2000).

Educable children have the right to eight years of free education, and children who are considered trainable receive healthcare and rehabilitation services. The maximum age of registration in the first grade of the elementary school for a student with intellectual disability is thirteen years. There are minimal opportunities for disabled adults for work and for care (Samadi, 2008). Critical issues for people who have disabilities are access to inclusive education, providing early intervention based on community-based rehabilitation methods, and employing adults who have disability in Iran (Samadi, 2008).

The medical model applies to the case study of Sarah from Iran, who is a fifteen-year-old female student in Grade 7. In this model, disability is considered as a problem with the mind and/or body and results in limited functioning that is seen as limited and deficient. A feature of this model is the trust of specialized professionals for diagnosing and treating conditions. The educational context for this group of children typically involves segregated special education classrooms within residential or live-in schools (Palmer & Harley, 2012).

As in the following narrative, even though Sarah's mom did not want to separate her daughter from her peers, and even though Sarah's exclusion from public school combined with the inaccessibility of even specialized schools caused some problems for her, she did not have any other options.

According to Blustein (2012), the medical model suggests that, like in Sarah's case, the built environment and societal organization do not give individuals with disabilities the same opportunities as those who are seen as typically functioning. The medical model suggests that problems faced by individuals with disabilities are independent of sociocultural, physical, or political environments: they are focused on what is seen as individual impairment (Brittain, 2004). According to Sarah's parents, Sarah has not received any community support.

SARAH'S STORY

Today is the first day of the new school week, and I am hoping to see Sarah at school. Last week, Sarah was absent for the whole week. Her mom called and let the school know that Sarah's dad was not home, and she did not have a ride to school. Sending her by taxi would be very expensive as her home is far from our school. The inaccessibility of special schools, like ours, can compel parents of children with disabilities to enroll their children in schools that are far from home. These types of schools in Iran are limited. For instance, in Tehran, the capital city of Iran with a population of around 8.7 million and an area of 751 square kilometers, there are only 52 special schools in total.

Sarah is in Grade 7, I thought to myself, but she is supposed to be in Grade 9. She had started school at age eight, two years later than most students. Her mom explained to me that it was a shock for her to learn that her daughter could not attend the local public schools. When Sarah was six years old, her mom and dad had taken her to register for Grade 1 at a public school near their home. She was sent there for regular health assessment, as students in Iran need to do a general health assessment before starting school. Some centers in Iran do this kind of examination. The centers examine physical and mental wellness, such as monitoring dental health, vision, hearing, weight, and IQ. If there is a mental or physical health issue, children will be sent for more examination at a related center.

One of the regulations for registration at public schools in Iran is that students must obtain adequate scores on a medical assessment based on an IQ test to see whether a child is considered educable. Students who score under 70 are considered in need of a special school. Sarah's score on this test was below the average. The medical personnel then told Sarah's parents that Sarah has an intellectual disability called mental retardation and needs to

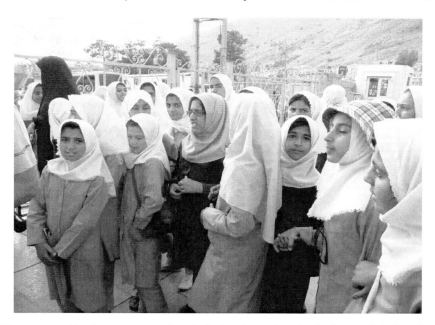

Figure 10.1 Youth in Iran may face inclusion issues in schools due to their learning profile. Case Story #10. *Pixabay License.* https://pixabay.com/photos/iran-school-class -girl-651311/.

attend a segregated or "special" school, since the speed of learning in children with intellectual disabilities is slower than the average. According to Iranian deputy minister of Prevention of the Welfare Organization (2018), birth rates of mental retardation infants in Iran due to consanguineous marriages are higher than the world average.

Sarah's mom found it to be a struggle for her to accept her daughter's situation. At first, she thought she might be able to teach her daughter at home. After two years of trying, she was unsuccessful due to her lack of experience in this field, so eventually she did send her to a special school. Fortunately, there were not any issues with her registration for Grade 1 at a special school, even though she was eight years old. Children in the same grade might have different ages at special schools as children can start elementary school at the age of six, and the highest age for entrance to high schools is twenty-two years.

Every day, when Sarah goes to school, the vice-principal guides her to the class, and her special education teacher and teaching assistant greet her before Sarah even sits on her chair. Being away from school for one week, for students in Sarah's situation, means a lot of additional work. However, this is a situation that they are familiar with and have some strategies to prevent students from being behind the rest of the class, such as a home-school communication booklet for parents to have some ideas about strategies they can use at home. Teaching in a special school is flexible, according to each student's level. Also, having a limited number of students in each class and hiring teachers' assistants are also helpful strategies so that Sarah's teacher is able to spend more time with those students who need more practice.

BRIEF CRITICAL RESPONSE QUESTIONS

1. Do you think medical personnel should determine the type of the schools and benefits for individuals without attention each individual's values and wants?
2. Discuss the advantages and disadvantages of exclusion of children with disability from public schools for both children with disabilities and neurotypical children.
3. Explain how you would help the parents of students who have not accepted their child's situation to understand the need to attend a special school?

REFLECTIVE RESPONSE QUESTIONS

1. Sarah had been absent for one week. What strategies do you recommend her parents using at home to prevent her from being behind her schedule?
2. What strategies would prevent her from being behind the group after she returns to class after her absence?
3. In Sarah's situation where education is not easily accessible, do you think online education might be a solution? Discuss its positive and negative points.

STRATEGY OF SUPPORT TO CONSIDER

- Inclusive programs and having children with special needs in the same school that typically developed children attend can decrease mental pressure on parents and make destinations closer.
- Having some home-school communication book can help those absent from school do not feel they are behind others.

CONCLUSION

This narrative presents the story of a girl from Iran who has excluded from public schools because of her disability. The Iranian educational system for children with disabilities follows the medical model, and children with disabilities are required to complete their education at segregated special schools. The inaccessibility of special school buildings made the commuting between home and school difficult for children with disabilities. Inaccessibility to community support made the situation of this group of children more difficult.

LINK TO THE RELEVANT ONLINE MATERIAL/VIDEO

- Mental Health Innovation Network https://www.mhinnovation.net/innovations/school-health-implementation-network-eastern-mediterranean-region-shine
- "Just like other Kids" https://www.hrw.org/sites/default/files/report_pdf/iran1019_web.pdf

REFERENCES

Bigdeli, M. R. (2000). Children rights and disabled children rights at international level. *Research Institute of Exceptional Children.*

Blustein, J. (2012). Philosophical and ethical issues in disability. *Journal of Moral Philosophy, 9*, 573–587. https://doi.org/10.1163/17455243-00904002.

Brittain, I. (2004). Perceptions of disability and their impact upon involvement in sport for people with disabilities at all levels. *Journal of Sport & Social Issues, 28*, 429–452. https://doi.org/10.1177/0193723504268729.

Exceptional Children Education Organization. (2020). *Exceptional children.* https://exceptionalchildren.org/project2020.

Grossman, H. J. (Ed.). (1983). *Classification in mental retardation.* American Association on Mental Retardation.

Iranian Deputy Minister of Prevention of the Welfare Organization. (2018). *Welfare organization guide: Birth rates for mentally retarded children in Iran are higher than the global average.* https://www.hrw.org/report/2018/06/27/i-am-equally-human/discrimination-and-lack-accessibility-people-disabilities-iran#.

Palmer, M., & Harley, D. (2012). Models and measurement in disability: An international review. *Health Policy and Planning, 27*, 357–364. https://doi.org/10.1093/heapol/czr047.

Roush, S. E., & Sharby, N. (2011). Disability reconsidered: The paradox of physical therapy. *Physical Therapy, 91*, 1715–1727. https://doi.org/10.2522/ptj.20100389.

Samadi, S. A. (2008). Comparative policy brief: Status of intellectual disabilities in the Islamic Republic of Iran. *Journal of Policy and Practice in Intellectual Disabilities, 5*(2), 129–132. https://doi.org/10.1111/j.1741-1130.2008.00160.x.

Chapter 11

Case Story #11—How to Strengthen a Child's Vulnerability by Providing Support at School?

Case Story from Croatia

Sanja Skočić Mihić, Zorica Janković,
Sanja Tatalović Vorkapić, and
Snježana Sekušak Galešev

This case study brings an international perspective on mental health–related needs of a student presented within two school settings of a Croatian educational context. The case study of Marko—male, age 15, Grade K-9, special classroom, regular school—is a firsthand narrative from a school professional associate who is certified as a psychotherapist. The first part of this narrative story is focused on the description of environmental factors that shaped social interaction in the elementary school setting. The second component depicts school staff members in the promotion of mental health and well-being. The application of effective, supportive, and nurturing interventions that shape the environment in addressing mental health issues in the context of Bronfenbrenner's (1998) bioecological theory of development is highlighted.

THEORETICAL MODEL AND BACKGROUND

Croatian educational system has undergone transition in line with social and economic changes during last thirty years of independence of the Republic of Croatia. As a small democratic parliamentary republic, known as a low- and mid-income country in European Union, Croatia went from postwar reconstruction, thought social reforms, and democratization to economic development. Still faces different aspects of family and social instability. The most relevant social issues connected to economy are unemployment (8.6 percent comparing to average 7.2 percent in EU), risk of poverty, single family, and rate of 1/3 divorces (Šućur et al., 2015; Novak et al., 2020; Croatian Bureau of Statistics, 2018).

Barry et al. (2013) stated that mental health in low and middle-income countries is a neglected public issue. Even though the mental health is one of the main domains within the National Health Strategy in Croatia, it seems more on declarative than proactive level. There is no universal, evidence-based prevention program in our country that would serve to strengthening all basic aspects of mental health in children and youth. Especially, when the focus is on children with special needs. There are numerous early intervention and prevention MH programs, various according their content, activities, and methodologies, mostly not scientifically evaluated. Some of them (various Erasmus+ projects' activities) are still in the phases of application and evaluation.

According to National Office for Drug Abuse Prevention of Croatia (http://www.programi.uredzadroge.hr/), there are 262 educational programs in Croatia that are aimed to promote children's mental health. However, only seventy-nine of them are applied at educational institutions, such as kindergartens, primary and secondary schools. In kindergartens (for children aged from six months to six/seven years), three programs are designed for preschool children, two for their parents and one for preschool teachers. In primary schools (children aged from six/seven to thirteen/fourteen years), thirty programs are designed for primary school children, eleven for their parents and one for primary school teachers. Finally, in secondary schools (children aged from fourteen/fifteen to eighteen/nineteen years), twenty-four programs are created for secondary school students, six for their parents and one for secondary school teachers. Educational institutions are free to choose between various MH programs what will be applied each school year in their kindergarten/school, and there is no national coordination between educational institutions regarding MH programs applications.

The high-quality epidemiological data of mental health issues and intervention in Croatia are scarce (Novak et al., 2020). According to epidemiological national survey, one-third Croatian children and youth experienced "some form of physical abuse combined with other violent act" (Ajduković et al., 2012, p. 401), and more them 35 percent experienced peer violence (Sušac et al., 2016). Multiple victimization and vulnerability in childhood is common and highly predictive factor of child trauma (Ajduković et al., 2012).

Bronfenbrenner's bioecological theory (Bronfenbrenner & Morris, 1998), which was upgraded to the ecological theory of development (Bronfenbrenner, 1979), was chosen to conceptualize the integrated human development through ecology theory within the Process–Person–Context–Time (PPCT) model. Examining the ecology of human development involves interrelated components of human development individual into the context as well as biological, cognitive, emotional, and behavioral characteristics, and the context of human development and time (Bronfenbrenner, 1979).

According to Bronfenbrenner's theory, human development starts from biology through ecology. In other words, the features of the developing person are influenced by external context that is described on five levels: micro, meso, exo, macro, and chronosystem. The smallest and most immediate microsystem involves personal relationships with family members, classmates and teachers and has the strongest impact on human development. The child's inner and out worlds are "fused and dynamically interactive" (Bronfenbrenner, 1979) and their relationships with others are parts of larger, enmeshed systems at multiple levels (Lerner et al., 2002). Therefore, nurturing and supportive interactions and relationships play crucial roles in building healthy child development, positive mental health and wellbeing, resilience, personal capacity and life skills, and academic and social outcomes.

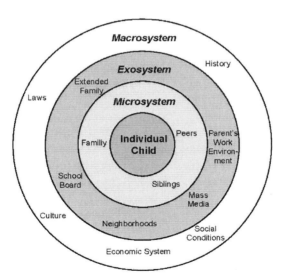

Figure 11.1 Bioecological model. Adapted from Halsall, T. et al. (2018). Case Story #11. *Examining integrated youth services using the bioecological model: Alignments and opportunities.* International Journal of Integrated Care. 18*(4)*. http://doi.org/10.5334/ijic .4165. https://www.researchgate.net/figure/Bronfenbrenners-Ecological-Model-displaying -the-multiple-contextual-levels-Original_fig1_329326124.

As Eriksson et al. (2018) pointed out, this theoretical framework can be used for explanation and promotion of mental health by considering interactions between environment context and personal characteristics.

Adaptive cognitive functioning, positive self-esteem, problem-solving skills, skills to cope with life changes and stress, and skills in shaping the environment are personal factors that contribute to well-being or positive mental health (Jané-Llopis et al., 2005).

As an integral part of overall health, mental health is "an individual's capacity to lead a fulfilling life including the ability to form and maintain relationships, to study" (WHO, 2013, p. 7) and refer to the equilibrium of the individual and the environment determinants. As Lavikainen et al. (2000) state: (1) individual factors and experiences such as childhood events, emotions, cognitions, self-esteem, autonomy, adaptive capacities, resilience; (2) social interactions such as personal and family sphere, school, services; (3) societal structures and resources such as educational resources, availability and quality of services; and (4) cultural values such as societal value given to mental health, rules regulating social interactions, social criteria of mental health, stigma, and tolerance, are determinate of individual mental health.

In the past two decades, the concept of mental health promotion is rising within a global political agenda (European Communities, 2005) and positive mental health and well-being are recognized "as fundamental to the quality of life and productivity" (Jané-Llopis, 2007, p. 191). In order to enhance competencies and reduce inequalities, the collaborative delivery of effective intervention and programs can help to achieve positive mental health (Jané-Llopis et al., 2005). According to Ottawa Charter (WHO, 1986), creating a supportive environment is one of five components of evidence of the efficacy of interventions for mental health promotion and a means to create schools as supportive environments for children to learn and grow (Jané-Llopis et al., 2005). Schools are a major setting for mental health promotion, including a large proportion of students, and enabling social networks, friendships, and school connectedness: the latter being a key protective factor for positive mental health (e.g., Jané-Llopis & Berry, 2005). As Rossen and Cowan (2014) pointed out that we should be aware that many children enter school with temporary or permanently mental health issues such as "bullying, deployment, divorce, death, illness, poverty, community violence, homelessness, abuse, or chronic mental illness such as depression, generalized anxiety disorder, and emotional-behavioral disorders" (pp. 8–9).

So, "the promotion of positive mental health must also be an integral part of the school ethos" (Jané-Llopis & Berry, 2005). Along with effective interventions in the mental health promotion in schools, contemporary interventions are effective across diverse groups and across the lifespan, including comprehensive programs that target multiple health outcomes in the context of a coordinated, whole-school approach (Antolić & Novak, 2016; Mrazek & Haggerty, 1994; O'Connell et al., 2009) or combine the school curriculum, pupils' knowledge and skills, the school ethos and environment, and involve the parents and the local community (e.g., Barry et al., 2013; Lukić Cesarik, 2012). Contemporary interventions promote positive mental health, and quality of life, and contribute to the reduction of mental health issues.

Teachers and other school staff members have a unique position to recognize the wide range of mental health issues. They are aware of their role in supporting the mental health among students in their schools and willing to participate in mental health education programs, while they feel moderately confident to deal with mental health issues (Reinke et al., 2011; Graham et al., 2011). Namely, teacher preparation during pre- and in-service education is not adequate to respond to diverse mental health issues and circumstances, and their "assumptions, values, beliefs, and attitudes about children's mental health" are linked to "their confidence and skill in supporting children's social and emotional well-being" (Graham et al., 2011, p. 479; Muslić, 2018).

Reinke et al. (2011) found that teachers perceive mental health promotion more in the psychologist's domain than teachers. So, they perceive the implementation of classroom-based behavioral interventions is in the teacher domain while teaching socio-emotional lessons, prevention and intervention of mental health in school such as screening, behavioral assessments, intervention and monitoring and referring to community services are in psychologist area.

In responding to challenges that students face in the school context, such as social exclusion, teachers have a unique opportunity for a prompt reaction that encourages and actualize student potential (Rak, 2012). Primary, shaping a positive classroom climate will reduce inappropriate behaviors such as aggression and bullying.

Bullying is specific harmful behavior that occurs in and out of school settings. It means the use of aggressive behavior systematically with an intention to harm a weaker peer who is not able to defend himself by different levels of physical, verbal, and/or psychological violence (Monks et al., 2009). According to international studies (WHO, 2012), 13 percent of students from eleven to thirteen years have suffered from bullying.

It is always an unequal relationship of power and strength that influence children and adolescents' healthy development with short and medium-term, or lifelong effects (Navarro et al., 2015). These effects harm the quality of life of children and adolescents including their physical and social well-being. It is fast becoming a worldwide public health problem (WHO, 2012). Research showed that witnessing social bullying would result in increased social anxiety and depressive symptoms (Fitzpatrick & Bussey, 2010), victims reported a higher level of depression, social anxiety, social isolation, school phobia, psychosomatic symptoms, low self-esteem (Barchia & Bussey, 2010; Mazzone et al., 2018). Therefore, prevention of bullying is vital in classrooms by creating positive school experiences that significantly influence positive behavior and development and strengthen academic and socio-emotional abilities. Orchestrating a positive classroom environment is a demanding and complex task for teachers, which necessarily involves collaborating with parents and other professionals both within and outside of school settings.

Family circumstances shape students' behavior, and family strengths and functioning, and the presence of psychosocial stressors in family and school settings should be recognized as a baseline in planning effective intervention to provide maximum support.

It should be pointed out that the complexity of school settings can influence children's development in many different ways. Within the case of Marko, following and according to the Process–Person–Context–Time (PPCT) model, the impact of the elementary school environment on Marko's development can be monitored. The higher quality of Marko's well-being in high school, as seen from his behaviors and reported by parents, is influenced by external school context on levels of micro and mesosystems. The interaction between the supportive environment and Marko's socio-emotional development over time is evident.

MARKO'S STORY

Marko has long-time record of developmental disabilities and was formally diagnosed with a behavior and emotional disorder as well as a speech disorder since K–1. He had an IEP that included curriculum modifications from K–3 only. He is an only child; his mother works and his father retired early due to post-traumatic stress disorder (PTSD). (He had participated in the Croatian homeland as a defender during 1991–1995). His parents shared a detailed narrative of Marko's experience through his school history.

After he finished primary school, Marko completed a professional program at an authorized agency and received a recommendation to enroll in a three-year program for an auxiliary administration occupation in line with Level 3 of European Qualifications Framework (EQF). The program is within a regular high school of economics through partial inclusion, which means that most subjects he has in the special classroom of four students. Several subjects are in special classrooms of ten students and one subject was within a regular class of twenty-four children. Here is some background information during K–1 and K–8:

According to his fathers' report, Marko was joyful and social included with peers during the preschool and K–1 grades. At the beginning K–2, though, a new student came into the class and started bullying him. Marko complained to his father that other boys were ignoring him, kicking him out of the game, and insulting him (e.g., "What is that jerk going to do with us?"). Later on, Marko began to report to his father that the boys were physically bullying him (e.g., hitting him into the stomach). Marko was also exposed to social isolation. For example, no one in the class wanted to talk to him, his peers didn't return his greeting, they pushed him out of line, no one wanted to sit with him at school nor on a bus trip. In higher grades, those experiences became worse. They posted porn photos on him and wrapped photos around his head. After his absence due to illness, the other boys kicked him out of classroom telling him that he is not supposed to go to the elective subject of computer science, although he was not enrolled in computer science classes. After that, he no longer wanted to attend computer science classes and dropped out. Then he became even more socially isolated and started to hide in the toilets and wait for teachers to find him.

At that time, he recounted to his father in detail all the experiences at school. His father, in turn, always responded to Marko's painful experiences by seeking support from teachers. After witnessing no change in support, his parents addressed Marko's harmful experiences with the school psychologists, and later, to the school principal and even with the parents of other students. But the father claimed that the school staff did not carry out any intervention around Marko's calls for help. He explicitly cited the words of one school staff members who said: "We should not interfere in children's affairs." While the school situation became even worse, Marko started running away from school and hiding, and, when he was extremely stressed, he started to have behavioral outbursts such verbal and physical aggression toward his parents. After Marko was included in the intensive and individualized intervention program, however, of a newly employed school psychologist during his K–8 years, his father reported a positive impact on Marko's behavior and well-being: started going to school more easily and happily, improved his academic achievement, and his verbal and physical aggression at home was reduced.

BACKGROUND INFORMATION: K–9

During his first contact with a psychotherapist, Marko showed himself to be a nice and gentle student, both withdrawn and timid. In the classroom setting, he behaved in a way that made him seem almost absent and very difficult to reach. He found it difficult to verbalize his current feelings or feelings from previous situations. He responded only when asked or prompted and answered questions only briefly. He didn't carry his cell phone even though he had one. At that point, he had no friends from elementary school or from the neighborhood.

Marko arrived at the school every morning at 7:45 am in the van for students with disabilities. According to his admission procedures, a school assistant welcomed him in front of the school door at the ground floor with greetings: "Marko, how are you?" Marko would not respond verbally and turned his head to the side. But he uttered swear words, used offensive language, changed his usual speaking voice tone to sound threatening and intimidating, ignored other school staff and students, and walked to the classroom on the first floor. Entering the classroom, he sat at his school desk in a hunched posture sideways facing the exit, refused to open his school bag of books, and looked to the side to avoid eye contact with his teacher or other students. One peer came to him and tapped him on his shoulder saying, "Come on, the teacher is coming!" Marko told him: "Get away from me," and pushed him away. The teacher entered the class and insisted that Marko take out his books, but when Marko didn't respond to the request, his teacher took his books out of his bag, placed them on the school table. Marko threw them off the table, cursing.

The school special teacher with school staff analyzed the situation. It was clear that these situations happened in the days when Marko gets out of the van and rolls a white piece of paper in his hands. The special teacher made a safety plan for Marko for situations that were demanding, such as running out of class, throwing books off of the table, and not responding to staff requests.

The next day, Marko arrived at the school and the assistant noticed that he was rolling a white paper in his hands. Therefore, the assistant did not greet him and did not look at him. Marko walked calmly to the classroom and sat down at the table. When Marko was ready, he showed interest and was actively involved in the teaching process. Then, teachers asked questions and gave him appropriate tasks that he could solve, activities to participate in, and opportunities to build his self-esteem.

The school team has worked hard to recognize Marko's triggers and to put into place some coping strategies such as not disturbing him in the classroom in order to allow him to self-regulate and creating a home-school communication plan with his parents. It was then evident that Marko enjoyed classroom activities such as practicing math and word puzzles, listening to music, celebrating his and his peers' birthdays. He prefers social interaction in his small classroom of ten students and participating in individual interventions with the specialized teacher who is also licensed as psychotherapist, where he has an opportunity to talk about ideas that he enjoys and is treated with respect.

BRIEF CRITICAL RESPONSE QUESTIONS

1. Analyze the opportunities in school setting K1–8 and K–9 for socio-emotional development?
2. Browse through interventions that the teacher can organize to promote positive behavior and acceptance of diversity for students.
3. What suggestions can be made to Marko's parents?
4. Address the Determinants of Positive Mental Health in K–9.

REFLECTIVE RESPONSE QUESTIONS

1. Imagine that Marko was five years old and analyzed the elements from his narrative story that could have been nurturing and supportive. List the types of interactions and relationships that have been provided to Marko in line with Bronfenbrenner's model and put them in relation to possible outcomes?
2. The main topic of Markos's story is focused on how environmental factors contributed to mental health issues? Explain the concept of mental health promotion and teacher responsibility?
3. Name and describe two of Markos's behaviors that reflect a need for additional support in mental health issues. Support your choices. Rationalize your choices with support from peer-reviewed literature.
4. Explain the intervention in K9 that you could improve on in order to enhance Markos's social outcomes. List the interventions that you may disagree with.
5. Reflect on the impact of primary school experiences on Markos's academic achievement and school curriculum. He is very good at math. His math teacher compares his ability with students in regular four years administration programs. What does this information point to? How have you perceived Marko's strength in accordance with available support?
6. Markos's father wrote a letter of thanks to the ministry highlighting that his current school is the example of how a school setting is able to effectively respond to individual student needs. How can you explain that Markos's misbehavior at home is reduced and he is happily going to school?

STRATEGIES OF SUPPORT TO CONSIDER

- greater awareness for mental health issues and education of school staff about positive mental health

- a wholistic approach to students' academic and socio-emotional development
- school staff need to work on positive school climate that promotes mental health
- provide school staff with professional service and networks and share resources
- *"on-going collaboration with the interprofessional team (i.e., administrators, classroom teacher, special education teacher, school behaviour teaching assistant, social worker, psychoeducational consultant, community agencies, family, medical practitioners)"*
- teacher higher level of competencies in coordinating curriculum and socio-emotional development toward lifelong-orientated skills and social outcomes
- establish intervention plan to respond to student needs and collaborative approach
- maximize students' educational achievement and well-being through partnership with parents and parental active participation
- available professional support to parents

LINKS TO RELEVANT ONLINE MATERIALS

1. Promoting Mental Health in Schools: https://www.promehs.org/

CONCLUSION

In this case study, using an authentic narrative, one can observe all continuum approaches from ignorant to supportive to needs of a vulnerable student. A few key points that emphasize the role of school in promoting mental health are presented: the way how difficulties can be interpreted, how classroom experience shapes development, how school staff is educated and collaborate in the promotion of mental health, how parent's enrolment is a constituent part of student well-being.

The case study starts from Bronfenbrenner's bioecological theoretical model that described human development as a process of person that is happening in context through time and the concept of mental health promotion in school settings. Through real-life case contexts school staff approaches to mental health can be viewed in continuum from the perspective out of sight, problem-focused interpretation and lack of understanding in K1–8, toward caring, supportive, and empathetic approach in K–9, that bring hope to student and parents.

The school staff collaboration and collaboration with parents in K–9 emphasize an appreciative, positive, and strength-focused school approach that provide better student outcomes. This narrative which covers a longer period of schooling brings valuable contribution to the comprehension of theoretical and research knowledge to teachers, school staff, and other holders of teacher education. We hope that prospective teachers and current teachers will have a unique opportunity to learn: (1) the importance of experience in the school environment to enhance students' well-being, regardless of developmental difficulty, but precisely because it is particularly important; (2) new ideas, strategies, and intervention to support and advocate the student in classroom; and (3) the importance of collaboration between school staff that provide a comprehensive approach to students need and partnership with parents.

The distinctive contribution of this story is in presenting a case study that depicts many relevant elements of mental health care in the Croatian school system and places itself in an international perspective. It can be concluded that this personal story of the student and his parents, which they selflessly presented for the purposes of this case, should be viewed as a resource to encourage significant and systematic changes in mental health promotion in the Croatian education system respecting individual needs of each student and his strengths in building inclusive societies.

To conclude, the mental health promotion and provision of intervention in school is extremely important for varied vulnerable groups of children, and is the role and responsibility of people working across a range of sectors, based on student need and right to receive appropriate support to ensure school and life skills and achievement (Rossen & Cowan, 2014).

REFERENCES

Ajduković, M., Rimac, I., Rajter, M., & Sušac, N. (2012). Epidemiološko istraživanje prevalencije i incidencije nasilja nad djecom u obitelji u Hrvatskoj. *Ljetopis socijalnog rada, 19*(3), 367–412. Preuzeto s https://hrcak.srce.hr/96677.

Antolić, B., & Novak, M. (2016). Promocija mentalnog zdravlja: Temeljni koncepti i smjernice za roditeljske i školske programe (Promotion of mental health: Basic Concepts and program guidelines for parental and school settings. In Croatian). *Psihologijske teme, 25*(2), 317–339. https://hrcak.srce.hr/161868.

Barchia, K., & Bussey, K. (2010). The psychological impact of peer victimization: Exploring social-cognitive mediators of depression. *Journal of Adolescence, 33*(5), 615–623. https://doi.org/10.1016/j.adolescence.2009.12.002.

Barry, M. M., Clarke, A. M., Jenkins, R., & Patel, V. (2013). A systematic review of the effectiveness of mental health promotion interventions for young people in low and middle income countries. *BMC Public Health, 13*(1), 835. https://doi.org/10.1186/1471-2458-13-835.

Bronfenbrenner, U. (1979). *The ecology of human development: Experiments by nature and design.* Harvard University Press.

Bronfenbrenner, U., & Morris, P. A. (1998). The ecology of developmental processes. In W. Damon & R. M. Lerner (Eds), *Handbook of child psychology: Theoretical models of human development* (pp. 993–1028). John Wiley & Sons Inc.

Croatian Bureau of Statistics. (2018). Statistical yearbook. *Zagreb: Croatian Bureau of Statistics*. https://www.dzs.hr/Hrv_Eng/ljetopis/2018/sljh2018.pdf.

Eriksson, M., Ghazinour, M., & Hammarström, A. (2018). Different uses of Bronfenbrenner's ecological theory in public mental health research: What is their value for guiding public mental health policy and practice? *Social Theory & Health, 16*(4), 414–433. https://doi.org/10.1057/s41285-018-0065-6.

European Communities. (2005). *Green paper: Improving the mental health of the population: Towards a strategy on mental health for the European Union.* Luxembourg (LUX): EC. https://ec.europa.eu/health/ph_determinants/life_style/mental/green_paper/mental_gp_en.pdf.

Fitzpatrick, S., & Bussey, K. (2010). The development of the Social Bullying Involvement Scales. *Aggressive Behavior, 37*(2), 177–192. https://doi.org/10.1002/ab.20379.

Graham, A., Phelps, R., Maddison, C., & Fitzgerald, R. (2011). Supporting children's mental health in schools: Teacher views. *Teachers and Teaching, 17*(4), 479–496. https://doi.org/10.1080/13540602.2011.580525.

Hrvatski zavod za javno zdravstvo – programi. http://www.programi.uredzadroge.hr/.

Jané-Llopis, E. (2007). Mental health promotion: Concepts and strategies for reaching the population. *Health Promotion Journal of Australia, 18*(3), 191–197. https://doi.org/10.1071/HE07191.

Jané-Llopis, E., & Barry, M. M. (2005). What makes mental health promotion effective? *Promotion & Education, 2*, 47–55, 64, 70. https://doi.org/10.1177/10253823050120020108.

Jané-Llopis, E., Barry, M. M., Hosman, C., & Patel, V. (2005). Mental health promotion works: A review. *Promotion & Education, 12*(2), 9–25. https://doi.org/10.1177/10253823050120020103x.

Lavikainen, J., Lahtinen, E., & Lehtinen, V. (2000). Public health approach on mental health in Europe. *National Research and Development Centre for Welfare and Health, STAKES Ministry of Social Affairs and Health.* https://www.julkari.fi/bitstream/handle/10024/75893/public2.pdf?sequence=1.

Lerner, R. M., Rothbaum, F., Boulos, S., & Castellino, D. R. (2002). Developmental systems perspective on parenting. In M. H. Bornstein (Ed.), *Handbook of parenting: Biology and ecology of parenting* (pp. 315–344). Lawrence Erlbaum Associates Publishers. https://psycnet.apa.org/record/2002-02628-011.

Lukić Cesarik, B. (2012). Psihološka procjena i rana intervencija kod djece i mladih s poteškoćama u razvoju uz podršku njihovim obiteljima. In V. Božičević, S. Brlas, & M. Gulin (Eds), *Psihologija u zaštiti mentalnog zdravlja: Priručnik za psihološku djelatnost u zaštiti i promicanju mentalnog zdravlja* (pp. 138–147). Zavod za javno zdravstvo "Sveti Rok" Virovitičko-podravske županije.

Mazzone, A., Nocentini, A., & Menesini, E. (2018). Bullying and peer violence among children and adolescents in residential care settings: A review of the literature. *Aggression and Violent Behavior, 38*, 101–112. https://doi.org/10.1016 /j.avb.2017.12.004.

Monks, C. P., Smith, P. K., Naylor, P., Barter, C., Ireland, J. L., & Coine, I. (2009). Bullying in different contexts: Commonalities, differences and the role of theory. *Aggression & Violent Behavior, 14*, 146–156. https://doi.org/10.1016/j.avb.2009 .01.004.

Mrazek, P., & Haggerty, R. J. (1994). *Reducing risks for mental disorders: Frontiers for preventive intervention research.* National Academy Press.

Muslić, L. (ur.), Markelić, M., Vulić-Prtorić, A., Ivasović, V., & Jovičić Burić, D. (2018). *Zdravstvena pismenost odgojno-obrazovnih djelatnika u području mentalnoga zdravlja djece i mladih. Istraživanje prepoznavanja depresivnosti i spremnosti na pružanje podrške i pomoći, Zagreb: Hrvatski zavod za javno zdravstvo, 2018 (prirucnik).* https://www.hzjz.hr/wp-content/uploads/2018/10/Zdravstvena -pismenost_publikacija.pdf.

Navarro, R., Ruiz-Oliva, R., Larranaga, E., & Yubero, S. (2015). The impact of cyberbullying and social bullying on optimism, global and school-related happiness and life satisfaction among 10–12-year-old school children. *Applied Research Quality Life, 10*, 15–36. https://doi.org/10.1007/s11482-013-9292-0.

Novak, M., Parr, N. J., Ferić, M., Mihić, J., & Kranželić, V. (2020). Positive youth development in Croatia: School and family factors associated with mental health of Croatian adolescents. *Frontiers in Psychology, 11*, 611169. https://doi.org/10 .3389/fpsyg.2020.611169.

O'Connell, M. E., Boat, T., & Warner, K. E. (2009). *Preventing mental, emotional, and behavioral disorders among young people: Progress and possibilities.* National Academy Press. https://doi.org/10.17226/12480.

Olsson, C. A., Bond, L., Burns, J. M., Vella-Brodrick, D. A., & Sawyer, S. M. (2003). Adolescent resilience: A concept analysis. *Journal of Adolescence, 26*, 1–11. https://doi.org/10.1016/S0140-1971(02)00118-5.

Rak, V. (2012). Unaprjeđivanje kvalitete psihosocijalnog okruženja i potpore učenicima u školi: iskustvene preporuke i upute za rad psihologa. In V. Božičević, S. Brlas, & M. Gulin (Eds), *Psihologija u zaštiti mentalnog zdravlja: Priručnik za psihološku djelatnost u zaštiti i promicanju mentalnog zdravlja* (pp. 101–108). Zavod za javno zdravstvo "Sveti Rok" Virovitičko-podravske županije.

Reinke, W. M., Stormont, M., Herman, K. C., Puri, R., & Goel, N. (2011). Supporting children's mental health in schools: Teacher perceptions of needs, roles, and barriers. *School Psychology Quarterly, 26*(1), 1–13. https://doi.org/10.1037/a0022714.

Rossen, E., & Cowan, K. C. (2014). Improving mental health in schools. *Phi Delta Kappan, 96*(4), 8–13. https://doi.org/10.1177/0031721714561438.

Šućur, Z., Kletečki Radović, M., Družić Ljubotina, O., & Babić, Z. (2015). *Siromaštvo i dobrobit djece Predškolske Dobi u Republici Hrvatskoj.* Ured UNICEF-a za Hrvatsku.

Sušac, N., Ajduković, M., & Rimac, I. (2016). Učestalost vršnjačkog nasilja s obzirom na obilježja adolescenata i doživljeno nasilje u obitelji [The frequency of peer violence with respect to characteristics of adolescents and experienced violence in the family]. *Psihologijske teme, 25*, 197–221. https://hrcak.srce.hr/161862.

World Health Organization (WHO). (2012). *Health behaviour in school-aged children (HBSC) international report from the 2009/2010 survey. In social determinants of health and well-being among young people.* http://www.euro.who.int/_ _data/assets/pdf_file/0003/163857/Social-determinants-of-health-and-well-being -among-young-people.pdf.
World Health Organization (WHO). (2013). *Investing in mental health: Evidence for action.* https://apps.who.int/iris/handle/10665/87232.

Chapter 12

Case Story #12—Trauma and School Supports in the United States

Erika Brindopke and Meaghan McCollow

THEORETICAL MODEL AND BACKGROUND

The following case study follows Iosefina, a fifteen-year-old, grade-10 student in the Counseling Enriched Classroom (CEC) at an urban comprehensive high school in Northern California in the United States. Within California, the CEC (sometimes called an Intensive Counseling Enriched classroom) is a setting used to support learners who have a history of significant trauma, including abuse and neglect, and present with emotional and behavioral issues that indicate more intensive supports are needed. In some cases, learners placed in a CEC are transitioning back to a public school setting from a nonpublic school setting (i.e., a specialized school for learners with exceptional needs that cannot be met in a public school setting). In the United States, the Individuals with Disabilities Education Act (IDEA) is the US Department of Education law governing special education across the country. While each state may interpret portions of the law differently, there are principles that are held across the United States. One such principle is called Least Restrictive Environment (LRE). LRE mandates that learners should only be in placements that are as restrictive as necessary. That is, that a learner should not be placed in a setting that is more limiting than their support needs indicate. Most frequently, LRE is viewed as a spectrum, with one side being the general education classroom with little or no supports and the other side being a specialized setting, typically outside of a public school setting. The CEC functions as a separate classroom from general education classrooms but is located in a public school setting. The model is to embed mental health counselors into the CEC to support academic and/or social success of learners. Mental health counselors work collaboratively with school staff to create a supportive, trauma-informed learning environment.

Erika Brindopke and Meaghan McCollow

In this CEC, the model of practice combines evidence-based practices of behavior modification and therapy, trauma-focused cognitive behavioral therapy, motivational interviewing, solution-focused therapy, dialectical behavior therapy, social learning therapy, and harm reduction. Learners may spend all or part of their day in this CEC, depending on individual goals as determined by their Individualized Education Plans (IEP). Learners in this classroom have qualified to receive services under the IDEA disability category of "Emotional Disturbance," which is a large category that may include individuals who have been diagnosed with anxiety, depression, PTSD, attention deficit hyperactivity disorder (ADHD), obsessive compulsive disorder (OCD), and so on. Many learners have comorbid diagnoses, such as autism spectrum disorder and PTSD, anxiety and depression, and so on. The CEC of focus in this case includes a special education teacher, a licensed therapist (Licensed Clinical Social Worker; LCSW) assigned to the classroom, two mental health counselors (i.e., not licensed therapists or social workers, minimum requirement is a bachelor's degree for this role), and up to thirteen high school students (this varies across the day, depending on the subject and learners' academic goals). This CEC is often referred to as the "Seneca classroom," as there is a partnership between the school district and the nonprofit organization called Seneca Family of

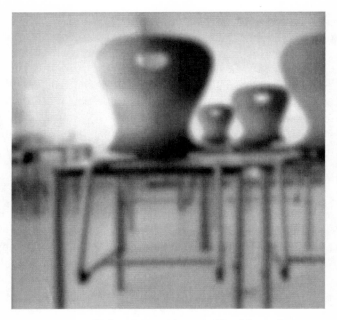

Figure 12.1   Inter-connected classroom with mental health services. Case Story #12.
Pixabay License. https://pixabay.com/illustrations/man-student-chair-lockdown-school
-6819496/.

Agencies. Seneca Family of Agencies provides the mental health services in the classroom, while the district helps fund the agency.

Iosefina joined the CEC at the end of her freshman year of high school. At the point in which the narrative takes place, Iosefina is spending four class periods—out of six across the day—in the CEC. These class periods include basic history, basic English, basic math, and basic science. Iosefina has a history of receiving special education services. She was first diagnosed with a speech/language impairment at the age of seven and began receiving special education services at that time. At about age ten, she was reclassified as eligible for services under the category of specific learning disability. Then, at about age fourteen, she was again reclassified to receive services under the category of emotional disturbance. Her ninth grade year began with Iosefina moving from one high school to another to yet another. Iosefina experienced various traumas prior to her placement in the CEC of focus in this case study, including homelessness, placements in group homes, and other domestic violence situations.

IOSEFINA'S STORY

Objective

It is my first day working at a comprehensive public school, I am a new mental health counselor in the CEC on campus. I make my rounds in the classroom, individually introducing myself to each student. When I walked over to Iosefina's desk, her head was down on her desk, I introduced myself, "Hi, my name is Ms. Erika, I'll be working here as a mental health counselor, what's your name?" Her hair was draping over her face as she looked up to whisper, "Iosefina."

Iosefina missed the majority of the first semester of her sophomore year due to hospitalizations surrounding her safety and the safety of her siblings. Due to these conflicts at home, Iosefina relocated to a residential program for a few months during that first semester of her sophomore year. When she returned to the CEC, it was already the second semester of her sophomore year. Having spent little to no time with her since we had met, it was time to start building rapport with her. There were plenty of times in the classroom where she would sit quietly at her desk, head down, writing in her journal. During class time, it appeared as though she was writing notes on the topic that the teacher was explaining; however, when approaching her desk, I noticed instead of writing notes she was writing song lyrics. When her teacher would call on her to answer a question, she would wear a blank stare on her face and shrug, saying, "I don't know."

There were many days like this where she would seem as though she was in her own world, unaware of what was going on externally, but attempting to cope with whatever feelings were coming up internally through writing in her journal. Whenever I would approach her and ask if she wanted to check in or talk, she would decline and shake her head no. The classroom therapist and I started to brainstorm how we could build trust with her, in order to meet her at her level and encourage her to express her thoughts and feelings. Since writing in her journal seemed to be a release for her, we decided to try passing notes to Iosefina. Instead of verbally asking her what was wrong or how she was feeling, I wrote those questions on a piece of paper and passed it to her. It was as though we opened a locked door. Iosefina began writing how she was feeling and proceeded to answer follow-up questions through writing. Through this process, Iosefina slowly started communicating her needs with staff more frequently. The majority of the emotions coming up for her were feelings of anger and irritation related to conflicts she was having either with siblings or peers. She often became triggered in her mainstream classes because students yelling at one another reminded her of moments of violence she experienced at home within her family. When Ioseinfa was triggered in these moments, she would leave class without permission and find a quiet place to hide.

One time when peers arguing in class triggered her in mainstream class, she left the class and hid inside of a stall with a sharp object in the girl's

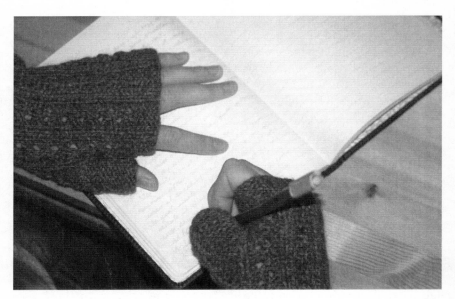

Figure 12.2 Journal writing as a form of reflection. Case Story #12. *Pixabay License.* https://pixabay.com/images/id-360791/.

bathroom. It took a team, including myself, an administrator, and a security guard to negotiate with Iosefina and encourage her to come out. Several incidents, including this one, led me to create a behavioral contract with Iosefina. The purpose of the behavioral contract was to support her in managing her difficult emotions of anger and irritation in a safe way. When Iosefina communicated her need to engage in a positive coping skill, such as writing, drawing, or walking to a trusted adult in the classroom, she earned a signature on her contract. Once she earned twenty signatures, she decided her reward would be a lunch out with classroom staff.

BRIEF CRITICAL RESPONSE QUESTIONS

1. Browse online information on internalized behaviors. What kinds of behaviors come up in your search? What strategies for supporting learners exhibiting those behaviors can you find?
2. How might you support Iosefina in finding a safe or quiet space to go to in moments that bring up past traumas? How might you support Iosefina in accessing that space safely and with responsible adults knowing where she is?
3. Find and describe an example of a behavioral contract that might be used with students who have similar characteristics to Iosefina.

REFLECTIVE RESPONSE QUESTIONS

1. Iosefina's counselors and teacher were able to build a trusting relationship through patience and finding her interests. What other strategies would you use to develop trust and respect with Iosefina? Support your answer.
2. Name, describe, and explain two or three components of a behavioral contract you would include in Iosefina's contract. Rationalize the inclusion of those components through peer-reviewed literature.
3. How would you communicate with Iosefina's teachers her needs related to removing herself from a classroom space during a trauma episode? What information would you provide her teachers to rationalize supporting Iosefina in the classroom?
4. A trauma-informed classroom practice assumes that learners bring with them their lived experiences. Conduct a brief literature search to find peer-reviewed articles focused on creating a classroom environment that incorporates trauma-informed practices.

5. Many learners carry trauma that educators may or may not be aware of. What might be the benefits of incorporating trauma-informed practices into any classroom, at any level? Focus on a grade level that is relevant to you and describe how educators might incorporate these practices, supporting your response with peer-reviewed literature.

Strategies of support to consider:

- Use of positive behavioral intervention supports in the classroom
- Creating a learning environment that promotes safety, rather than stress
- Utilizing restorative justice in place of punitive punishments like suspensions
- Incorporate trauma-informed teaching tools in the classroom
- Strengthening the students' relationships with teachers/support staff, as well as increasing their trust in school

LINKS TO RELEVANT ONLINE MATERIALS

- Anderson, E. M., Blitz, L. V., & Saastamoinen, M. (2015). Exploring a school-university model for professional development with classroom staff: Teaching trauma-informed approaches. *School Community Journal*, *25*(2), 113–134. https://files.eric.ed.gov/fulltext/EJ1085667.pdf.
- Crosby, S. D. (2015). An ecological perspective on emerging trauma-informed teaching practices. *Children & Schools*, *37*(4), 223–230. https://doi.org/10.1093/cs/cdv027.
- Crosby, S. D., Howell, P., & Thomas, S. (2018). Social justice education through trauma-informed teaching. *Middle School Journal*, *49*(4), 15–23. https://doi.org/10.1080/00940771.2018.1488470.
- Emdin, C. (2016). *For White folks who teach in the hood... and the rest of y'all too: Reality pedagogy and urban education.* Beacon Press.
- Jennings, P. A. (2018). *The trauma-sensitive classroom: Building resilience with compassionate teaching.* WW Norton & Company.
- Morris, M. W. (2019). *Sing a rhythm, dance a blues: Education for the liberation of black and brown girls.* The New Press.
- Reinke, W. M., Herman, K. C., & Stormont, M. (2012). Classroom-level positive behavior supports in schools implementing SW-PBIS: Identifying areas for enhancement. *Journal of Positive Behavior Interventions*, *15*(1), 39–50. https://doi.org/10.1177/1098300712459079.

REFERENCES

Anderson, E. M., Blitz, L. V., & Saastamoinen, M. (2015).Exploring a school-university model for professional development with classroom staff: Teaching trauma-informed approaches. *School Community Journal, 25*(2), 113–134. https://files.eric.ed.gov/fulltext/EJ1085667.pdf.

Crosby, S. D. (2015). An ecological perspective on emerging trauma-informed teaching practices. *Children & Schools, 37*(4), 223–230. https://doi.org/10.1093/cs/cdv027.

Crosby, S. D., Howell, P., & Thomas, S. (2018). Social justice education through trauma-informed teaching. *Middle School Journal, 49*(4), 15–23. https://doi.org/10.1093/cs/cdv027.

Emdin, C. (2016). *For White folks who teach in the hood... and the rest of y'all too: Reality pedagogy and urban education.* Beacon Press.

Jennings, P. A. (2018). *The trauma-sensitive classroom: Building resilience with compassionate teaching.* WW Norton & Company.

Morris, M. W. (2019). *Sing a rhythm, dance a blues: Education for the liberation of black and brown girls.* The New Press.

Reinke, W. M., Herman, K. C., & Stormont, M. (2012). Classroom-level positive behavior supports in schools implementing SW-PBIS: Identifying areas for enhancement. *Journal of Positive Behavior Interventions, 15*(1), 39–50. https://doi.org/10.1177/1098300712459079.

Chapter 13

Case Story #13—Despite the Best of Intentions

A Case of Mental Health in a Fragile Context in Haiti

Steve Sider and Samuel Charles

THEORETICAL MODEL AND BACKGROUND

On January 12, 2010, the land of Haiti literally shook. Thousands were killed, and hundreds of thousands were left with even less than the meager belongings that they had just hours earlier. Many schools were destroyed or severely damaged. It is estimated that the earthquake destroyed or badly damaged nearly 5,000 schools and killed approximately 38,000 students and 1,300 teachers (Leeder, 2010). Across the country, those schools that were not damaged remained closed for many months. In April 2010, schools outside of Port au Prince began to open. To understand Haiti's educational system after the earthquake, the context for this case, one must have an awareness of the context of education in Haiti.

In Haiti's first constitution of 1805, universal primary education was declared and Haiti became the first country in the world to guarantee access to education for all. Yet, 200 years later, universal access to education has not occurred in Haiti. Approximately 77 percent of children in Haiti attend primary schools and less than 30 percent attend secondary school (UNICEF, 2020). Further, those who do attend school tend to attend low fee private schools with only approximately 15 percent of students attending the public school system (Sider et al., 2019). The educational context is significantly influenced by economic and political challenges of Haiti.

Haiti is considered the poorest country in the Western Hemisphere and one of the poorest in the world with a gross domestic product (GDP) per person of $846 (World Bank, 2020). Nearly 60 percent of the population survives on

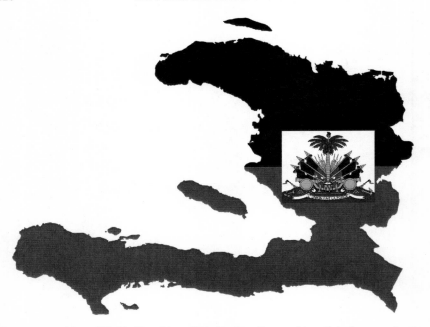

Figure 13.1   Map of Haiti. Case Story #13. *Pixabay License.* https://pixabay.com/vectors
/haiti-flag-map-borders-country-5323242/.

less than $2.50 per day (World Bank, 2020). As a result, often families will
send one child to school since they cannot afford the fees that accompany
school enrolment even in public schools (Sider et al., 2019). As well, children
may not go to school because they need to supplement the family income
(Rice et al., 2016).

Due to the challenging economic situation, there are limited financial
resources to support education and mental health resources in Haiti. Haiti's
fragile political structure leads to weak governance of the education and
health systems. Corruption and nepotism have been documented in public
life in Haiti (Ramachandran & Walz, 2015). Money that could be spent on
supporting education and mental health resources is often spent on other
priorities or disappears from the public purse altogether. Further, societal
norms intersect with the provision of mental health supports. For example,
in Haitian schools, students with mental health concerns are often bullied
and experience corporal punishment at the hands of school administrators
(Nicolas et al., 2012). They are often marginalized in school or expelled
from it. There are very limited mental health resources in Haiti so mental
illnesses are often undiagnosed, and most teachers have no training in mental wellness (Nicolas et al., 2012). It is within this context that we describe
our case.

CASE STORY

In 2010, Alec Morvan (all names are pseudonyms) was a Grade-10 student at LekendyMetulus High School in Cap-Haitien, a city of half a million people in Haiti's north. LekendyMetulus High School was a large public high school. It accommodated two shifts of students: 3,000 came in the morning from 8:00 am to noon and then another 3,000 students attended from 1:00 pm to 5:00 pm. It is common in urban areas in Haiti to have such an arrangement where limited resources and an increasing demand for education have led to overpopulated and under-resourced schools. There are often 80–110 students per class in these schools. Despite the challenges of such an educational context, Alec had demonstrated himself to be a student leader respected by his peers and the teachers. Although he had grown up in a family with very limited financial means, his parents had made every effort to ensure that Alex and his sisters were able to attend school. All three children had flourished in school and were strong leaders, providing a model for others who had experienced similar hardships.

Like many other schools in the country, LekendyMetulus High School welcomed students from Port au Prince to finish the school year after the 2010 earthquake. Despite being a six-hour drive north of Port au Prince, Cap-Haitien was a common destination for students from Port au Prince after the earthquake since it was the country's second largest city and many students had relatives there. Alec's Grade 10 class welcomed three new students who had experienced the earthquake in Port au Prince. Alec was president of his class council and felt a responsibility to ensure the students' integration into the new school. Alec had made significant strides to build a supportive school structure where the 1,500 or so students in his grade had engaged in community-building efforts such as supporting local children's programs, clean-up days, and assisting those with disabilities. Alec was confident that he and his classmates could effectively support the inclusion of the new students into the school.

One of the new students particularly caught everyone's attention. Jean-Pierre was seventeen years old and was from Delmas, a section of Port au Prince. His father had died when Jean-Pierre was a child and he lost his mother and a younger brother in the earthquake. He also mourned the death of several of his uncles, aunts, cousins, and friends in the earthquake and he himself barely escaped death as his house collapsed in front of him. Jean-Pierre had been a strong student in his previous high school in Delmas and was optimistic about pursuing postsecondary studies to be an engineer. The 2010 earthquake significantly changed his demeanor. He had experienced the devastating loss of both his parents, a sibling, and many relatives and friends. Now, just a few months later, he found himself living with a distant relative in a city he had never been to before.

Alec made himself available to Jean-Pierre and the others who had just arrived. When they first arrived at LekendyMetulus High School, Alec was one of the first to greet them and to let them know that he was available if they needed anything. Alec had developed a document that provided some of the community outreach programs that he and his classmates were involved in and he shared this with the three new students. It was quickly evident that Jean-Pierre wanted to keep his distance from everyone and did not respond to Alec's overtures of friendship or invitation to be involved in the community-building events. Of course, no one had any idea what he had gone through during the earthquake.

One Thursday, just a week after the three new students had arrived, Alec was going to his class on the first level of the high school. As he approached the entrance to the classroom, he noticed an argument involving Jean-Pierre and another student. When Alec intervened and asked what was happening, he was told that Jean-Pierre had sat in the seat assigned to the other student. When the student demanded his seat, Jean-Pierre refused. Despite Alec's intervention, the tension escalated quickly and the two got into a physical fight. A teacher came running to the scene and both students ended up at the principal's office.

Leaving the school that afternoon, Jean-Pierre was in tears. Alec heard him cry out, "I've got no place in this rotten school or in this city!" He then hurled some insults directly at students who were hanging around the school, one of whom was Alec. Before Alec could respond, Jean-Pierre ran off in the direction of where he was living.

The next day Jean-Pierre did not come to class and his absence was noticed, initially by Alec and the other students. Of course, the teachers did not notice since it was almost impossible for a teacher to notice the absence of a student when there were 100 or 120 students in the same classroom. Alec did not pay much attention to the fact that Jean-Pierre was absent; it was not an uncommon thing since students often also had to find ways to support their families while enrolled in school.

The next Monday, Jean-Pierre was back in the class. Alec went to talk with him and to let him know that it was not necessary to fight with other students for a seat. Alec told him that he could talk with the teacher and arrange for Jean-Pierre to have a seat in the class for the rest of the year. He was about to invite Jean-Pierre to a community event that he was leading that evening but was interrupted by Jean-Pierre: "Why don't you leave me alone? I hate this place and I hate you. I don't care about this community so why would I even do something to support it?"

Jean-Pierre's reaction shocked Alec. Jean-Pierre angrily told Alec that he could fend for himself and that Alec should mind his own business. Alec stood there as Jean-Pierre walked away. Alec thought to himself, *What can I do now? He clearly does not want my help and he's so angry.* Alec mulled it over but did not know what to do to support Jean-Pierre.

Later that week, a student saw Jean-Pierre covertly drinking alcohol in class before the teacher arrived. The student told Jean-Pierre that it was against the school regulations and that he could get into serious trouble if he got caught. Jean-Pierre made it clear that he did not care about the rules. The same day, while in a literature class, Jean-Pierre was invited to answer a question. He responded with a sarcastic tone in his voice: "I don't see why we're wasting precious time studying people who have died." The teacher was not pleased with the response. He asked Jean-Pierre to leave the room immediately, but he refused because, in his opinion, he had done nothing wrong. The teacher left the room to seek help from the principal. Even when the principal accompanied the teacher, Jean-Pierre still refused to leave the classroom. After about thirty minutes, he was forcibly removed from the classroom and taken to the principal's office. Jean-Pierre was punished with a strap, a form of corporal punishment which is an unpleasant reality of school life in many schools in Haiti.

After school, Jean-Pierre waited for the teacher outside the entrance of the school. He was angry and he verbally attacked the teacher as Alec watched in shock, Jean-Pierre appeared to be ready to physically assault the teacher. It was the first time the students had seen a student confront a teacher like that and the students were stunned. Alec and a number of others quickly got between Jean-Pierre and the teacher. Alec tried to remain calm as he escorted Jean-Pierre away from the scene. Within seconds, Jean-Pierre ran away. The teacher was clearly stunned by the confrontation. The next day, Alec found out that Jean-Pierre had been permanently expelled from the high school.

CRITICAL QUESTIONS

1. What similarities and differences would you note between students such as Alec and Jean-Pierre in Haiti and students within your own context?
2. Why might Jean-Pierre have responded as he did in different parts of this case?
3. What strengths-based perspectives and assets did Alec bring to this case?
4. In what ways can students and staff work collaboratively to build healthy school communities in fragile contexts?
5. Identify a context that could be considered fragile or challenging and which has developed a strengths-based, school-based framework to support mental health. What are the key aspects of the initiative? How was it developed despite the challenges of the context? Could it be adapted for other contexts?

REFLECTIVE RESPONSE QUESTIONS

1. Jean-Pierre arrives at your high school for the first day after experiencing multiple tragedies during his lifetime, most recently a massive earthquake that has killed many of his family and friends. Describe a short- and long-term process of mental health support that you would advocate for.
2. As a teacher or principal of LekendyMetulus High School, how would you prepare the students and teachers in the school to best support students who were being introduced to the school after having experienced significant tragedy and relocation?
3. Although this case is situated in Haiti, what other country or regional examples can you identify that would have similar intakes of students who have experienced significant trauma? Engage in a brief inquiry to see if you can identify resources that organizations such as the UNICEF, Save the Children, or the Inter-Agency Network for Education in Emergencies have developed.
4. How might mental health supports be made available in culturally appropriate ways in fragile and financially constrained contexts or for students who are coming into your school from those contexts?
5. Engage in an inquiry to develop an understanding of the diversity of mental healthcare supports available to students in multiple countries. What commonalities and differences can you identify in these supports? How does this inform your understanding in your local context?

STRATEGIES OF SUPPORT TO CONSIDER

1. Peer-to-peer support: High school students often respond best to peer support. This can be difficult since peers might not have sufficient training. However, providing training in schools on being mentally healthy, supporting others who are struggling, and knowing where to turn for resources and support should be provided. Check out the resources on peer support available on the Mental Health Commission of Canada website (https://www.mentalhealthcommission.ca/English/what-we-do/recovery/peer-support).

   Particularly *Opening Minds* (https://www.mentalhealthcommission.ca/English/opening-minds).
2. Mental Health First Aid for Teachers: This program provides formal training in helping a person experiencing a mental health problem or a worsening of their mental health (https://www.mhfa.ca/). Also check out SafeTALK and ASIST suicide prevention training programs which may be available in your area.

3. Professional development for teachers: Teachers are often on the front lines of recognizing the signs of mental illness and proactively supporting mental health. They also need to be aware of ways to ensure the maintenance of their own mental well-being. Education offices at state, provincial, or local levels often have excellent documents to build awareness, for example, *Supporting Minds* in Ontario, Canada (http://www.edu.gov.on.ca/eng/document/reports/supportingminds.pdf). Also, check out programs offered by local universities such as Wilfrid Laurier University's Mental Health Issues in the Classroom certificate (https://www.wlu.ca/professional-development/office-of-professional-development/mental-health-issues-in-the-classroom/index.html).

4. Support to access community-based resources: There are many resources available in communities to support students' mental well-being. These include crisis help services including phone and text-based options as well as counseling services. Do a scan of local and regional organizations supporting student well-being such as Kids Help Phone (https://kidshelpphone.ca/).

5. Supports specific for second language learners: If students are new to the country and have experienced trauma in their previous country context, they may also require support in their mother tongue or a language they are familiar with. Consider resources such as from the American Psychological Association (https://www.apa.org/monitor/2015/03/immigrant-children) or highly accessible sources such as Edutopia (https://www.edutopia.org/article/helping-students-trauma-tragedy-grief-resources).

CONCLUSION

Jean-Pierre was a victim not only of the 2010 Haitian earthquake but of a failing school system. Before the tragedy of January 12, 2010, it is unlikely that any school in Haiti had access to mental health supports, particularly psychological or counseling assistance for students and teachers. From the work we have done in schools in different regions of Haiti, we have observed that this has not changed. There are only a few psychologists and other mental health professionals in the country and their services are only available through a fee structure, something beyond what the vast majority of the population can afford. Fortunately, organizations like Partners in Health (https://www.pih.org/programs/mental-health) and Mennonite Central Committee (https://mcc.org/stories/healing-emotional-pain-supporting-mental-health-haiti) are providing localized, grassroots supports. However, many Haitians—particularly young people—are highly at risk with limited access to resources.

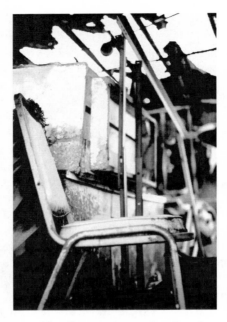

Figure 13.2   Schools ravaged by climate emergencies. Case Story #13. *Pixabay License.*
https://pixabay.com/photos/damaged-storm-flood-fire-5666668/.

In a context where there are limited financial resources, it is important to consider community-based and school-based supports that can be realized through teacher-led and student-to-student initiatives. These require less financial inputs and are nuanced to the needs of the local community. The work of the Inter-Agency Network for Education in Emergencies, International Health Policies, and UNICEF (see Resources) are helpful in developing these types of initiatives. We particularly would encourage those interested in this topic to consider the three-tier model that UNICEF has developed (see Resources). Although teachers in contexts such as Canada and the United States may not experience the type of natural disaster that Jean-Pierre experienced, they will have students in their classes who have been affected by these types of tragedies. Teachers—in countries as diverse as Haiti and Canada—are well served by developing their knowledge about mental health situations and supports that are reflected through this case.

RESOURCES

- Inter-agency Network for Education in Emergencies (2020). *Mental health and psychosocial considerations.* https://inee.org/resources/mental-health -and-psychosocial-considerations-during-covid-19-outbreak.

- International Development Agency (2020). *Overview of conflict and fragility.* https://ida.worldbank.org/node/411.
- International Health Policies (2019). *Mental health in conflict: The case of Yemen.* https://www.internationalhealthpolicies.org/featured-article/mental-health-in-conflict-the-case-of-yemen/.
- UNICEF (2020). *Community-based mental health and psychosocial support in humanitarian settings: Three tiered support for children and families.* https://www.unicef.org/media/52171/file.
- World Health Organization (2016). *Psychosocial support in fragile and conflict-affected settings.* https://www.worldbank.org/en/topic/fragilityconflictviolence/brief/psychosocial-support-in-fragile-and-conflict-affected-settings.
- World Bank (2016). *VIDEO: Making mental health a global development priority.* https://www.worldbank.org/en/news/video/2016/04/18/making-mental-health-a-global-development-priority.

REFERENCES

Leeder, J. (2010). Teaching without schools: Haiti after the earthquake. *Professionally Speaking.* http://professionallyspeaking.oct.ca/september_2010/features/haiti.aspx.

Nicolas, G., Jean-Jacques, R., & Wheatley, A. (2012). Mental health counseling in Haiti: Historical overview, current status, and plans for the future. *Journal of Black Psychology, 38*(4), 509–519. https://doi.org/10.1177/0095798412443162.

Ramachandran, V., & Walz, J. (2015). Haiti: Where has all the money gone? *Journal of Haitian Studies, 21*(1), 26–65. http://www.jstor.org/stable/24573148.

Rice, K., Girvin, H., Frank, J. M., & Corso, L. S. (2016). Utilizing expressive arts to explore educational goals among girls in Haiti. *Social Work With Groups, 39*(1), 1–14. https://doi.org/10.1080/01609513.2016.1258620.

Sider, S., Desir, C., Jean-Marie, G., & Watson, A. (2019). Exploring educational opportunities toward gender equity for girls in Haiti. In C. Sunal & K. Mutua (Eds), *Transforming public education in Africa, Caribbean, and Middle East.* Book Series: Educational Research in Africa, Caribbean, and Middle East. Charlotte, NC: Information Age Publishing. https://nsuworks.nova.edu/fse_facbooks/100.

UNICEF. (2020). *Haiti.* https://www.unicef.org/haiti/.

World Bank. (2020). *Haiti overview.* http://www.worldbank.org/en/country/haiti/overview.

About the Authors

Erin Keith, EdD, OCT

@DrErinKeith

Erin Keith is an award-winning assistant professor, Ontario certified teacher-leader, author, and research in inclusive education at St. Francis Xavier University (StFX), Nova Scotia, Canada. With a doctor of education degree in educational leadership from Western University, her own research focus centers on social justice issues related to investigating school-based mental health supports for students, and wellness literacy for teachers. This includes how to support children's mental health, self-regulation, social-emotional growth, and curating inquiry and wonder in inclusive, culturally responsive learning spaces. Erin is a passionate, wholistic educator, and a strong advocate for transformative teacher education programs using an asset and EDIDA lens—equity, diversity, inclusion, decolonization, and accessibility.

Kimberly Maich, PhD, OCT, BCBA-D, R Psych, C Psych

@KimberlyMaich

Kimberly Maich, is an award-winning professor, researcher, author, and clinician in inclusive education at Memorial University, Newfoundland and Labrador, Canada. She spent most of her early career as a resource teacher, supporting students with exceptionalities from kindergarten to Grade 12, as well as being a clinical coordinator with McMaster Children's Hospital's ASD School Support Program (Hamilton, ON) and tenured associate professor at Brock University (Niagara, ON). She is a special education specialist, a certified teacher, a registered / clinical psychologist, a full professor and Newfoundland and Labrador's first board certified behavior analyst (doctoral).

Manufactured by Amazon.ca
Acheson, AB

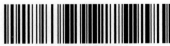

12106978R00088